HOPE IN THE HAZE: A DEMENTIA CAREGIVER GUIDE

PRACTICAL TECHNIQUES TO TACKLE CONFUSION, LIGHTEN EMOTIONAL BURDENS, AND EMPOWER YOU AND YOUR LOVED ONE TO THRIVE

CLARA LEON

CONTENTS

INTRODUCTION

I remember a rainy afternoon many years ago – the sort of classic gray drizzle that only Western Washington can deliver – and my feet were throbbing from hurrying between home visits. The sky loomed charcoal-gray as I stepped into the living room of a patient named Rita, who had moderate-stage dementia. She was staring at a family photo, her brow furrowed in puzzlement. Her daughter, Sandra, sat close by, rubbing Rita's back gently. When I came in, Sandra glanced at me with eyes that pleaded for answers. "Some days," she whispered, "it feels like I'm losing her piece by piece." That raw moment has stayed with me. It reflected the anguish so many caregivers endure, yet it also captured the deep devotion that propels them forward.

I've spent 25 years as a nurse caring for individuals with dementia. In that time, I've seen love and heartbreak woven together like a tattered quilt, each patch telling its own story. But I've also witnessed something extraordinary: the transformative power of knowledge, empathy, and a willingness to adapt. This book is meant to share that power with you.

A Purposeful Guide for Caregivers

My goal is to empower you—someone who may be juggling errands, family obligations, or work demands while caring for a loved one whose world is changing day by day. You might feel overwhelmed. You might worry about making mistakes or not having the right resources. That's understandable. Dementia can be unpredictable, tugging at the threads of memory, personality, and routine. But here's the truth: With the right guidance, you can shape a more supportive environment, safeguard your own well-being, and nurture a richer connection with the person in your care.

This book offers practical strategies: everything from modifying the home to reduce confusion, to handling legal and financial necessities, to safeguarding your own mental health. It also dives deeper, exploring communication approaches that preserve dignity and maintain emotional bonds. But it's not just about checklists. It's about forging a sense of community and compassion. Because, in many ways, caregivers stand at the front lines of compassion every single day.

Why Dementia Care Feels So Heavy

Worldwide, over 50 million people live with dementia—a number expected to triple by 2050. Behind each statistic lies a family grappling with heartbreak, exhaustion, and unknown challenges. The emotional toll alone can be staggering: watching a parent or spouse forget shared memories or seeing them struggle with once-familiar tasks. Physically, caregiving demands can leave you drained—lifting, bathing, cooking, cleaning, organizing medications. Logistically, it's a puzzle of appointments, insurance forms, and endless scheduling. And financially, it can be crippling. Many spend their life savings on specialized care or home modifications.

If you're reading this, you probably know these struggles firsthand. You may have had moments of panic, trying to keep your loved one safe during a wandering episode. Or perhaps you've felt pangs of guilt when frustration overtook your patience. I understand. I've watched patients slip into confusion during what used to be simple routines, and I've stood next to caregivers fighting back tears. But in that crucible of challenges, there's also the spark of humanity. A chance to rewrite the caregiving narrative so it's less about loss and more about growth, resourcefulness, and deepened love.

To You, the Caregiver

This book is for you. The one who wakes at odd hours to soothe anxieties or ensure a wandering loved one doesn't leave the house. The one who fights with insurance reps or hunts for a respite care program that fits a tight budget. The one who wonders if anyone else feels this alone. Let me assure you: You're not alone. There's an entire community of caregivers facing similar trials, and there's a network of professionals, neighbors, volunteers, and even technology waiting to support you. My aim is to stand beside you in these pages—to be that reassuring voice saying, "Yes, it's daunting, but you can do this. And there is help."

What This Book Covers

We'll start by unraveling dementia itself, separating myths from reality. Next, we'll discuss how to create a home that's safer and less confusing, focusing on everything from lighting to labeled cabinets. Then, we'll address communication, exploring strategies for validating your loved one's feelings, using gentle touch, or mastering the art of non-verbal cues. As the book progresses, we'll examine daily caregiving challenges—managing aggression or agitation, planning nutritious meals, organizing medications, and establishing consistent routines.

We'll also devote sections to legal and financial considerations, guiding you through topics like Power of Attorney, advanced directives, and finding financial resources for long-term care. Further along, we'll talk about self-care, exploring stress management, mindfulness, and building emotional resilience. We'll delve into the broad network of resources—support groups, community programs, digital forums, professional services—and showcase how tapping into them can lighten your load. And finally, you'll see how other caregivers overcame seemingly insurmountable hurdles, forging new identities and discovering moments of joy amidst the struggle.

What Makes This Book Different

Plenty of guides on dementia focus heavily on medical details or broad caregiver tips. This one blends my nurse's background with deeply personal insights I've collected over decades. Expect honest stories of heartbreak and triumph, practical checklists that don't shy away from real-life complexities, and emotional encouragement at every turn. We'll use real caregiver anecdotes to illuminate each chapter, weaving compassion and creativity throughout. Think of it as part manual, part memoir, part heartfelt conversation across your kitchen table.

The Path Ahead

Caregiving is rarely a straight line. It's more like a winding trail through ever-shifting terrain. You'll encounter obstacles you never foresaw. Good days can dissolve into chaos in minutes, and bad days can surprise you with a tender moment of clarity or love. My hope is that this book arms you with the knowledge to face the unexpected—both short-term solutions and long-term planning. You'll learn to adapt, to breathe through the hard moments, and to remain kind to yourself.

A quick heads-up: it's okay to feel uneasy. As we dive into topics like the decline of cognitive function or advanced planning for end-of-life care, you might feel a pang in your chest. That's normal. But facing these realities now grants a measure of control later. My promise is that we'll handle these subjects with empathy and respect, always respecting your courage and your loved one's dignity.

A Word of Encouragement

Before we start turning pages, I want you to pause. Look at your own resilience: the times you've soothed someone's tears, managed a tricky medication schedule, or coaxed a reluctant parent into a bath. Acknowledge how far you've come, even if you feel exhausted. That perseverance is already in you. This book merely builds upon it, providing tools and insights so you can care for your loved one—and yourself—with renewed confidence.

So, let's begin. Let's walk this road together, you and I. Let the next chapters remind you that each day, each frustration, each tiny victory, is part of a greater story of love. The journey won't be simple. But it can be profound, and it can bring meaning to moments that might otherwise slip away unnoticed. You have more strength than you know. This book is here to nurture that strength and guide you forward with hope.

A QUICK NOTE

In the pages that follow, you'll encounter personal stories drawn from my years of nursing experience. However, to respect the privacy and dignity of the families I've cared for, I've changed the names and slightly altered identifying details. The heart of their experiences remains the same—raw, honest, and transformative, just as I witnessed. By protecting their identities, we can focus on the universal truths of dementia caregiving and the compassion that binds us all.

UNDERSTANDING DEMENTIA AND ITS PROGRESSION

I remember the first time I encountered a family grappling with a dementia diagnosis. I was fresh out of nursing school, eager to help yet overwhelmed by the gravity of it all. The patient was a gentle man named Charles, who had once been known for his quick wit and fondness for crossword puzzles in The Seattle Times. His daughter, Rose, hovered at his bedside, insisting he was "just a little forgetful." She held onto this hope as if it were a lifeline. But I could see the trepidation in her eyes. The truth was painful: dementia isn't just a little forgetfulness. It's a life-altering shift in how the mind works, and for Charles, it marked the start of a journey that would challenge them both in ways they never expected.

Over the last 25 years, I've seen countless families walk this path. Some step forward with resolve, others with uncertainty, and many with both. No matter what, each story is different. Each person's mind unravels at its own pace and pattern. And each caregiver faces a delicate balancing act: offering support while preserving dignity. It's not easy, but understanding dementia —truly understanding it—can make all the difference.

In this chapter, we'll explore the basics of dementia, analyze its stages, and shine light on those early warning signs. We'll talk about the emotional toll it takes on families and the bewildering behaviors that so often accompany the disease. And finally, we'll map out a few ways to prepare for this journey so you can find solid footing in an ever-shifting landscape.

Take a deep breath. Let's begin.

THE BASICS OF DEMENTIA: SYMPTOMS AND CAUSES

Dementia vs. Normal Aging

Not too long ago, I cared for a proud woman named Yvonne who would stride into my clinic wearing bright turquoise sneakers. She insisted she was "just getting older" whenever she forgot where she placed her keys or stumbled over a friend's name. Many of us have moments like that. We walk into a room and forget why we're there, or we struggle to learn the latest phone app. That's normal aging. It might be frustrating, but it usually doesn't stop us from living our daily lives.

Dementia, however, is different. It's not merely losing your train of thought. It's walking into a familiar kitchen and not remembering which drawer holds the forks. It's forgetting entire experiences, people's names, or how to perform tasks you've done for decades. When these cognitive slips become so severe that they interrupt daily routines and personal independence, we're talking about dementia. This confusion often comes with changes in mood, language, and social behavior, painting a much bigger picture than simple forgetfulness.

Common Misconceptions

A frequent misconception is that dementia is a specific disease, like pneumonia or diabetes. Actually, "dementia" is more of a catch-all term. It describes a range of symptoms that stem from different types of brain disorders. Another myth is that it's exclusively a problem for "old people." While age is a big risk factor, younger individuals can develop early-onset forms too.

In my early days, I once thought that if someone spoke coherently, they couldn't have dementia. But I soon discovered patients who could hold polite, charming conversations while forgetting entire portions of their day. Dementia can be selective, unpredictable, and downright perplexing. Sometimes, you'll see clarity. Other times, confusion floods in.

Primary Causes and Types of Dementia

The top cause is Alzheimer's disease, accounting for roughly two-thirds to three-fourths of all dementia cases. Alzheimer's typically begins with subtle memory issues—like forgetting recent events—and escalates into significant language, problem-solving, and orientation deficits. Another form is vascular dementia, which often happens after a stroke. It arises from reduced blood flow to the brain. Sometimes, you'll see a blend of Alzheimer's and vascular dementia, complicating the picture even more.

Lewy body dementia is another major type. It can involve Parkinsonian features such as trembling or stiffness, plus vivid hallucinations. I once cared for a patient, Mr. Li, who sometimes saw unfamiliar people in his living room. He'd quietly offer them tea. He insisted they were real. It was heartbreaking yet enlightening to see how real these visions felt to him. There's also frontotemporal dementia, which may skew behavior and personality first, before memory takes a hit.

Causes: Genetic, Traumatic, and Lifestyle

Genetics do play a role. Certain gene variants can increase the risk of developing specific types of dementia. Still, having a genetic predisposition doesn't mean a diagnosis is certain. Brain injuries can also be culprits, from repeated concussions in athletes to a single severe trauma. And yes, lifestyle matters: factors like poor cardiovascular health, smoking, unmanaged diabetes, and lack of exercise can harm the brain over time.

Common Symptoms to Look For

- **Memory Loss**: Repeatedly asking the same questions or forgetting important dates.
- **Confusion**: Getting lost in a familiar place or not recognizing once-familiar faces.
- **Language Difficulties**: Struggling to find the right words or follow conversations.
- **Behavior Changes**: Sudden shifts in personality, irritability, depression, or anxiety.

Early Diagnosis Benefits

Spotting dementia early can make a world of difference. Treatments—while they don't cure—can slow symptom progression in some people.

Brain-stimulating activities, lifestyle adjustments, and certain medications can help. Early diagnosis also gives you time to plan, whether that involves setting up legal documents, seeking financial advice, or having meaningful conversations with your loved one about their wishes. I've seen families breathe a cautious sigh of relief when they finally name the struggle. That clarity, while scary, allows them to prepare and find support.

STAGES OF DEMENTIA: WHAT TO EXPECT

Dementia doesn't unfold the same for everyone. Some move through the stages slowly. Others advance rapidly. Still, it's helpful to have a roadmap.

Mild Cognitive Impairment (Early Stage)

Think of mild cognitive impairment (MCI) as the first warning bell. The changes are often small but noticeable. Maybe your loved one forgets appointments more often. Or you find an array of sticky notes around the house, reminding them to do everyday tasks. They can usually function mostly independently, but occasional slip-ups happen.

I recall a patient named Marianne. She was once a brilliant accountant, but she started mixing up numbers. She'd correct herself most of the time, but the errors grew more frequent. Her family said, "It's just stress," and Marianne nodded. Yet, deep down, she knew something was off. Over months, small mistakes snowballed. Finally, she sought help.

Moderate Dementia (Mid Stage)

Now the changes are more significant. The person needs help with daily activities: maybe meal preparation, bathing, or handling finances. A father might forget to turn off the stove after cooking lunch, or a mother might wander out of the house, unsure where she's heading. Behavioral changes can flare up. Anxiety, paranoia, or even aggression might appear. It's not that your loved one has turned mean—they're just confused, frightened, or frustrated. This is also where caregivers typically realize they can't do this alone, because the person's safety and well-being demand close oversight.

Severe Dementia (Late Stage)

In this final stage, the disease ravages memory, communication, and physical abilities. Many individuals can no longer speak in coherent sentences. Some become bedridden and dependent on round-the-clock care. It's heart-wrenching to watch. At this point, you may need professional care services or a skilled nursing facility's assistance. I've sat by many bedsides in this stage, holding hands that once were strong enough to lift children, now frail and unsteady. It's a time for compassion, tenderness, and preserving dignity.

The Progression Timeline

There's no set schedule. I've seen people remain in the mild stage for years, while others progress from mild to severe within a couple of short ones. Genetics, overall health, and environmental factors all play a role. Regular check-ups help track these changes. A doctor might adjust medications or recommend different therapies based on new behaviors or symptoms.

Medical Support Throughout the Journey

Staying connected to healthcare professionals is essential. Neurologists, geriatricians, therapists—they all bring unique perspectives. Check-ups allow you to share new concerns: "Mom seems more confused in the evenings," or "Dad isn't sleeping well." These updates help shape care plans. Remember, you're part of the care team. Your observations are invaluable.

A few years ago, I had a patient, Mr. Borden, who started sleeping all day. His wife dismissed it as normal aging, but I suspected something else. After consulting with his doctor, we discovered medication side effects were making him groggy. A small adjustment improved his alertness significantly. That's the power of staying vigilant and communicating openly with the care team.

RECOGNIZING DECLINE: EARLY SIGNS AND INTERVENTION

Spotting Subtle Shifts

It's easy to overlook early cognitive changes. People misplace keys or forget names all the time, right? Sure. But if these lapses become more frequent or severe—like forgetting entire events—pay close attention. Maybe your loved one suddenly struggles to follow a familiar recipe or handle a simple math problem. They might repeat stories in the same conversation, unaware they just told you that anecdote a minute ago.

A nurse colleague of mine, Patrice, once mentioned her uncle repeatedly telling the same childhood tale about a fishing trip. At first, the family laughed it off. But the repetition skyrocketed. He'd tell it three times in a single dinner. That was when alarm bells rang. It's these small, repetitive moments that often signal bigger issues beneath the surface.

Why Early Intervention Matters

Catching dementia early can't halt it. But it can slow progression, improve life quality, and give everyone time to adjust. Through therapy, medication, or lifestyle tweaks, many patients preserve mental function longer than they might have otherwise. Exercise routines, a healthier diet, and brain games—even crossword puzzles—can stimulate neural connections. More importantly, early intervention allows families to learn about resources, support groups, and coping strategies before they're in crisis mode.

Practical Strategies and Resources

- **Memory Enhancement Activities**: Simple card-matching games, puzzle books, or apps designed to challenge memory.
- **Support Groups**: Local community centers, hospitals, or online forums often host groups where caregivers and patients share stories, advice, and encouragement.
- **Counseling Services**: Professionals can guide both the person with dementia and their loved ones through tough emotional terrain.

Keeping a Cognitive Health Journal

Jot down notable changes. Did your spouse get lost driving somewhere familiar? Are they struggling with finances? Record dates and details. Bring these notes to doctor appointments. It provides a clear snapshot of their journey. I like to call it a "compassionate log" because it's not just data—it's the story of your loved one's day-to-day challenges. This helps professionals fine-tune interventions. It also validates what you're witnessing at home, so you're not second-guessing yourself.

THE EMOTIONAL IMPACT OF DEMENTIA ON FAMILIES

Common Emotional Reactions

Dementia is not just the patient's disease. It's the family's burden too.

When a person you love starts drifting away mentally, you might feel shock, denial, anger, sadness, even guilt. Some days you might feel all of these at once. I remember a daughter who broke down in tears, whispering, "I want my mom back." Another caregiver told me he resented the endless questions, then felt horrible for being upset. These emotions are natural. They don't make you a bad person. They make you human.

The Weight of Helplessness and Frustration

Helplessness can be the hardest emotion to bear. You can't stop the disorder. You can't wave a wand and restore what's slipping away. That often leads to frustration. You wish your loved one would just remember to lock the door, or you wish they wouldn't lash out when confused. But they can't help it, and neither can you. Accepting that helplessness can be strangely liberating. It allows you to focus on what you can do: providing comfort, support, and adapting their environment for safety.

Importance of Emotional Support for Caregivers

If there's one thing I've learned in my career, it's that caregivers often neglect their own well-being. They run themselves ragged trying to do it all. Don't. You need help. Therapy or counseling sessions can be a lifesaver. Family or friends might not always understand the depth of your stress, but a trained professional can. They'll offer coping strategies, a safe place to vent, and a reminder that you deserve to be cared for too.

Building a Support Network

Look around. Who can you lean on? Maybe a cousin who's willing to sit with your loved one while you grocery shop. Perhaps a neighbor who used to be a nurse. Or a friend who simply has a kind ear. Support groups—both in-person and online—allow you to connect with fellow caregivers who "get it." In these spaces, I've seen strangers become confidants. People share tips on everything from bathing techniques to navigating insurance. They also share tears, laughs, and successes. You don't have to do this alone.

Coping Strategies for Emotional Stress

- **Mindfulness**: A few minutes of deep breathing or guided meditation can bring calm amid chaos.

- **Self-Care**: Read a book, sip tea, or take a short walk. Even 15 minutes can recharge your mental battery.
- **Open Communication**: Talk to your family about your feelings. Have family meetings. Set boundaries. Don't let resentment fester in silence.
- **Realistic Expectations**: You can't fix everything. Identify what you can control and let go of the rest.

BEHAVIORAL CHANGES IN DEMENTIA: A DEEP DIVE

Aggression and Agitation

One of the most jarring parts of dementia is when a loving parent or spouse suddenly snaps at you. Imagine a gentle grandmother, always patient and kind, now yelling because she thinks someone stole her purse. Or a sweet old man who lashes out physically because he doesn't recognize his surroundings. This is heartache personified.

Early in my career, I cared for a retired teacher, Ms. Fuller, who once wrote poetry for fun. She started screaming at me because she was convinced her notebook had been stolen. In reality, it was right beside her. The outburst shook me. Later, I realized it was fear talking—fear of losing what little she had left. She was lashing out to regain control.

Repetitive Questioning and Confusion

"How do I turn on the TV?" your loved one might ask. You show them. Two minutes later, they ask again. Then again. Over and over. It can be maddening. But it's important to remember: they're not trying to annoy you. They genuinely can't recall what you just explained. Sometimes, confusion about time, place, or identity leads to repeated questions, seeking reassurance in a world that feels strange.

Why These Behaviors Occur

The neurological changes in dementia disrupt the brain's ability to process information. A memory that should stick simply doesn't. Imagine flipping through a photo album, but every time you turn a page, the previous photos vanish. That's their daily reality. Environmental triggers—like loud noises, crowded gatherings, or changes in routine—can exacerbate these behaviors.

• • •

Strategies for Managing Challenging Behaviors

- **Redirection**: Gently steer them toward something calming or familiar, like a family photo album or a favorite snack.
- **Structured Routines**: Predictability reduces anxiety. Keep meal times, bedtime, and activities as consistent as possible.
- **Calming Environments**: Soft lighting, gentle music, minimal clutter.
- **Patience & Empathy**: Take a breath before responding. Validate their feelings. "I see you're upset. Let's figure this out together."

The Power of Validation Therapy

Instead of arguing or correcting them—"Your purse isn't stolen!"—you acknowledge their emotion. "You're worried your purse is missing. That must be scary." Then you help them find it, or if it's right beside them, gently guide their eyes to it. That simple shift reduces confrontation and builds trust.

SETTING REALISTIC EXPECTATIONS

Recognizing Your Limits and Seeking Help

Caregivers often want to do everything. I once met a daughter, Lily, who insisted on caring for her father all by herself. She worked full-time, managed his meds, cooked meals, bathed him, and took care of her own kids. Eventually, she broke down in tears in my office. She was exhausted and felt guilty for being tired. "I should be able to handle this," she said. But none of us are superheroes. Seeking help—whether from family, professionals, or community resources—is a sign of wisdom, not weakness.

Flexibility and Adaptability

Change is inevitable. What works this month might fail next month. A friend of mine struggled with her mother's wandering. At first, a simple door alarm was enough. But as her mother's condition worsened, she learned to pick the lock. They adapted, installing more secure systems and placing motion sensors in the hallway. They also arranged a safe, fenced backyard for wandering. Each step was a response to a new development. Flexibility is key.

Long-Term Planning and Preparedness

Financial and legal preparations can seem daunting. But they're crucial. Setting up a power of attorney, drafting a will, or considering options like a trust can prevent chaos down the road. If your loved one is able, encourage them to express their wishes early. Talk about advanced directives, living wills, and care preferences. It might be uncomfortable, but it spares everyone from guesswork later.

Celebrating Small Victories

In the swirl of daily challenges, it's easy to focus on what's going wrong. But noticing even tiny successes can keep your spirits afloat. Maybe your loved one remembered where the coffee mugs were. Maybe they recognized a friend's voice. Or they had a day without outbursts. Celebrate that. Let these moments give you hope. Even in the advanced stages, there can be flickers of clarity or flashes of joy—a smile, a familiar joke, a snippet of an old song. They're precious.

A Personal Reflection

Sometimes, in the thick of it all, you might ask, "Is there anything good left?" I asked that once, years ago, during a night shift. A patient with moderate dementia kept calling out for her deceased husband. She wasn't frantic, but she was lost, searching for him. I sat by her side, holding her hand. When I reminded her that she had a daughter, she paused and said, "Yes, she's my sunshine." For a fleeting moment, there was love and warmth in her eyes, bright enough to chase away the darkness. We lose many things to dementia. But in those moments, we see what remains: the capacity to love, to feel safe, to share a spark of recognition. That's worth holding onto.

Final Thoughts

Dementia is complex. It changes minds, habits, and relationships. But knowledge is a powerful ally. By understanding the differences between dementia and normal aging, recognizing the range of possible causes, and spotting the early warning signs, you can approach care with clarity. Delving into the stages helps you anticipate what might come next, so each shift is less jarring. Realizing how deeply it affects not just your loved one but the entire family will guide you to seek emotional support, build networks, and practice self-care. And preparing for the journey with realistic expectations— knowing you can't do it all, that things will evolve, and that it's okay to ask for help—can sustain you through the toughest days.

You're not alone in this. Many have walked a similar path and found moments of grace, hope, and even joy. Yes, there will be heartbreak. There will be tears, arguments, sleepless nights, and days where confusion reigns. But there will also be moments of profound connection. A sudden flash of memory, a shared laugh, a gentle hand squeeze that says, "I'm still here, and I know you love me." Those moments can light up the most difficult road.

As you move forward, keep this in mind: caring for someone with dementia is not a sprint. It's a marathon that requires pacing, planning, and patience. It calls for empathy, creativity, and sometimes just a good sense of humor. Lean on your resources—medical professionals, friends, family, community organizations, support groups. Lean on hope, too. There's always room for that.

Remember the story of Charles and Rose. In the beginning, she insisted he was just aging. Then, as we delved deeper, she realized she needed help. Over time, she joined a support group, learned how to adapt his routine, and saw the difference a few changes could make. She found joy in hearing him hum an old tune from his youth. It's those little victories that add up. They aren't cures, but they are comforts.

And that's what we all need, isn't it? Comfort, knowledge, and under-standing. With them, this journey, while undeniably challenging, can also be filled with moments that remind us what it means to truly care for someone —mind, heart, and soul.

INTERACTIVE IDEAS WORTH CONSIDERING

- **Progression Timeline Chart**: Create a simple chart or calendar marking important milestones, doctor visits, and noticeable changes. This visual tool can help you track patterns and anticipate next steps.
- **Cognitive Health Journal**: Keep brief daily or weekly notes on your loved one's memory lapses, mood changes, and any interventions you try. This data is invaluable to share with healthcare providers.
- **Support System Checklist**: List friends, family members, neighbors, or community groups that can offer help, whether it's

cooking a meal, dropping by for company, or providing a break so you can rest.

- **Daily/Weekly/Monthly Checklist**: An organized checklist is a vital tool to help you stay proactive and maintain a structured approach in your caregiving journey. It guides you through essential daily tasks, encourages weekly reviews, and prompts you to evaluate monthly progress.

As you turn the page to the next chapter, hold onto the understanding you've gained here. Knowledge alone won't solve everything, but it can steady your footing and calm your heart. And here's a **bonus for you**: simply scan the QR code on this page to download your free daily/weekly/monthly checklist. Print it out, pin it to your fridge, tuck it into your caregiver note-book, or keep it handy on your device—just make sure it's always close by. Every little step counts as we move forward, one day at a time, one memory at a time, with compassion and courage lighting the way.

Scan the QR code on this page to download your free daily/weekly/monthly checklist

CREATING A DEMENTIA-FRIENDLY ENVIRONMENT

❦

I t's very common for me to walk into homes touched with dementia and find families wrestling with the condition. On one occasion, the patient's daughter had posted homemade signs all over the walls: "Kitchen," "Living Room," "Bathroom." She'd even labeled cupboards and drawers with pictures—cups, plates, spoons—everything carefully taped in place. The place looked a bit cluttered to me at first. But there was a warmth in that home. It was obvious she'd done these things out of love, hoping her father would find his way around a house that had become foreign to him. And in many ways, it worked. He stopped asking quite as often, "Where's the sugar, honey?" or "Which one's the bathroom?" That daughter's resourcefulness touched me deeply. It taught me that small modifications can turn a disorienting space into a familiar haven.

This chapter is an exploration of what it means to create a truly dementia-friendly environment. We'll talk safety. We'll discuss memory aids that can bring back a spark of recognition. We'll touch on how to handle wandering, a behavior that can be as frightening as it is common. Then, we'll dive into the technology that can lighten your load. And we'll end with a look at person-centered care and the power of community resources. Throughout these sections, I'll share stories and lessons from my decades as a nurse—stories of heartbreak, yes, but also of triumph and resilience.

DESIGNING A SAFE HOME: ESSENTIAL MODIFICATIONS

A Nurse's First Lesson in "Simple Fixes"

A few years into my career, I was called to the home of Margaret, a grandmother with early-stage dementia. Her son, Daniel, was frantic. She had slipped in the bathroom the week before, fortunately without breaking any bones, but it could have been far worse. When I arrived, I noticed that her shower floor was slick with no anti-slip mat. The bathroom rug was frayed and easy to trip on. There were no grab bars near the toilet or the tub. Daniel stood there with tears in his eyes, saying, "I can't believe I never thought about all this."

He wasn't alone in that oversight. Many caregivers don't realize how easily a common household fixture can become a hazard. Small changes can prevent major accidents. For Margaret, we started by installing a sturdy grab bar next to the toilet and another inside the shower. We replaced the old rug with a non-slip mat. Within a day, that bathroom was transformed from a hazard zone into a safer space. Daniel told me later, "I'm now sleeping better at night without worrying she'll break her hip." His relief was palpable.

Key Areas for Immediate Attention
Bathroom

- **Non-Slip Mats and Grab Bars**: A must-have. Put them in the shower, near the toilet, or anywhere your loved one steps in and out of the tub. These bars provide stability. They can literally be lifesavers.
- **Shower Seat**: If mobility is an issue, a simple shower chair can prevent fatigue and slipping.

Kitchen

- **Safe Storage for Hazardous Items**: Lock up knives, cleaning chemicals, or any item that could cause harm if used incorrectly. It's not about restricting independence but preventing accidents.
- **Stove Safety Knobs**: These can help avoid accidental gas leaks or burns. In some cases, you might even install an auto-shutoff device for electric or gas stoves.

Lighting and Visual Cues

Proper lighting does more than just brighten a room. It reduces confusion and disorientation. Imagine an older adult who wakes up at night, needs the bathroom, but can't find the switch in a dim hallway. That's a recipe for a nasty fall. So consider:

- **Motion-Sensor Lighting**: Hallways and bathrooms are prime locations for these. No fumbling for switches. No stepping into darkness.
- **Labeling**: As I saw in that home that I mentioned at the beginning of the chapter, labels on doors, cabinets, and even drawers can be magical. Large, clear words or pictures can guide someone who's struggling to remember what goes where.

You might feel like you're "baby-proofing" your house. And in a way, you are. Dementia can cause a person to lose familiarity with once-routine spaces. These cues can bring reassurance. I had one patient, Arthur, who always forgot which door led to the bedroom. His wife put a picture of a bed on the door, plus his name. Arthur would shuffle down the hall, see that sign, and break into a soft smile. "Ah, this is me," he'd say. That small sign changed his nightly routine from anxious wandering to a calm stroll toward rest.

Furniture and Layout Changes

When it comes to furnishings, minimalism can be a blessing. That doesn't mean you remove all the homey touches, but clutter creates hazards. A random stool in the middle of the living room might trip someone whose peripheral vision is failing or who's shuffling more than usual.

- **Remove Obstacles**: Keep pathways clear. If your loved one uses a walker or wheelchair, ensure wide, unobstructed paths.
- **Stable Furniture**: Chairs with armrests help seniors sit and stand more easily. Tables with rounded corners reduce injury risk if someone bumps into them.
- **Avoid Loose Rugs**: Even a small throw rug can send a person tumbling if it's not secured.

Routine Safety Checks

It's not enough to set up these modifications once and forget them. A home environment changes over time. New clutter appears. A grab bar might loosen. That's why monthly (or at least quarterly) safety evaluations matter.

- **Inspection Checklist**: Jot down items to check regularly: handrail stability, smoke alarm batteries, motion-sensor lights, loose wires.
- **Family Involvement**: Invite siblings, grandchildren, or neighbors to walk through the house with you. Fresh eyes might catch something you missed.

One caregiver, Harriet, told me she and her teenage son do a "safety sweep" every first Sunday of the month. They open every cabinet, scan for loose rugs, test the lights, and more. She said, "It's become our little ritual. And no doubt it's saved us from many close calls."

MEMORY AIDS AND TOOLS: ENHANCING DAILY LIVING

A Personal Story: The Power of a Simple Calendar

I once worked with a gentleman named David who, before his diagnosis, was a meticulous planner. He had a color-coded schedule for every part of his day. When dementia started creeping into his life, he grew frustrated. He'd forget doctor's appointments. He'd miss phone calls. His frustration sometimes spilled over into anger at himself—and occasionally at his wife.

I suggested they get a big whiteboard calendar and place it in their living room. Each morning, David and his wife would write down any appointments, mealtimes, or events. Over time, he found solace in that routine. He'd glance at the calendar, see his day neatly laid out, and feel more in control. That single tool reduced his anxiety significantly because it tapped into his old habit of structured scheduling.

Types of Memory Aids

- **Calendars & Planners**: Hang a large, easy-to-read calendar in a common area. If your loved one is comfortable with a smartphone, consider a shared digital calendar with reminders.
- **Labeling Systems**: For drawers, cabinets, or even the refrigerator. Simple words or images can guide daily tasks.
- **Checklists**: A to-do list for the day, checking items off as they're completed, can instill a sense of accomplishment.
- **Daily Exercises**: Crossword puzzles, word searches, or memory games. They keep the mind engaged.
- **Consistent Routines**: Doing the same tasks at the same time each day builds muscle memory and reduces confusion.
- **Repetition & Positive Reinforcement**: When they remember something successfully, praise them. Encourage that sense of victory.

One of my patients, Joanne, loved cooking. As her memory slipped, she started to forget recipes she'd made for decades. Her daughter laminated index cards with simple instructions for each dish—no more than five or six steps. Joanne used them daily, flipping through each step. It wasn't exactly how she used to cook, but it allowed her to keep doing what she loved, and that was priceless.

Visual and Auditory Reminders

Some folks respond better to hearing a reminder than seeing it written down. Others do better with visuals. Experiment:

- **Voice-Activated Devices**: "Alexa, remind me to take my pill at 9 AM." This has become a godsend for many caregivers.
- **Visual Schedules**: Print out a daily routine and stick it on the fridge. Add pictures or icons for each task (like a toothbrush for hygiene, a plate for mealtime).
- **Task Lists**: Step-by-step instructions near the stove, sink, or door. Keep them big and clear.

Personalization Matters

No two people are the same. A memory aid that works wonders for your neighbor's mother may baffle your dad. Tailor these tools to your loved one's preferences and history. If your dad spent a lifetime as a musician, maybe a short morning playlist triggers memories of simpler times. If your grandmother was a teacher, a mini chalkboard with notes might feel comforting and familiar.

My friend Elaine's father was an avid fisherman. In his bedroom, she hung pictures of fish species with big labels. Every morning, he'd wake up, see those pictures, and recall a bit of his old passion. Sometimes he'd share stories about "the big one that got away." That personal touch brightened his mood, reminding him that though some memories fade, others can still shine through.

MANAGING WANDERING: STRATEGIES FOR SAFETY

A Midnight Search That Changed Everything

I'll never forget the night I got a call at 1 AM from a panicked caregiver. Her husband, Jim, had slipped out the back door and wandered into the neighborhood. She found him two blocks away, standing in his pajamas, staring at a streetlamp. He was lost and disoriented but physically unharmed. The emotional toll on her was immediate and severe. She cried, "I was so scared he'd get hit by a car or freeze in the cold."

Wandering happens for many reasons: restlessness, confusion, a desire to "go home" even if they are home. It can be terrifying for caregivers who fear the worst every time their loved one steps outside.

Risks of Wandering & Prevention

- **Injury**: They might trip on uneven sidewalks or walk into traffic.
- **Exposure**: Inclement weather can be dangerous if they're dressed improperly.
- **Stress**: Both for the wanderer and for you, the caregiver, as you scramble to find them.
- **Door Alarms & Motion Sensors**: Simple systems that beep or send an alert if a door is opened during certain hours.
- **GPS Tracking Devices**: Worn like a watch or pendant. You can quickly locate someone if they roam.

- **Safety Locks**: Placing locks higher or lower than usual can deter someone who reflexively tries to open a door at a standard handle height.

I once met a family who installed a small chime on every exterior door. At first, they worried it might annoy them, chiming every time someone came or went. But they soon found the peace of mind far outweighed the mild inconvenience.

Reducing the Impulse to Wander

- **Structured Routines**: If your loved one has set times for walks, meals, and activities, they might feel less restless.
- **Engaging Activities**: Boredom can lead to wandering. Keeping hands and minds busy can diminish that urge.
- **Secured Outdoor Areas**: A fenced yard or a safe courtyard can allow someone to roam under controlled conditions.

An older gentleman I knew, Mr. Nelson, loved gardening. After he started wandering at night, his son built a small enclosed garden patch in the backyard. Each day, Mr. Nelson would spend hours tending plants, content in his little sanctuary. His nighttime wanderings lessened dramatically.

Emergency Response Plans

Despite best efforts, accidents happen. Prepare:

- **Emergency Contact List**: Family, neighbors, local police. Keep it visible on the fridge or next to the phone.
- **Recent Photo**: Have one ready to share if you need help locating your loved one.
- **Notify Authorities**: Some police departments have "Project Lifesaver" or similar programs designed to find missing seniors.

I recall a neighbor who informed the local fire and police station about her husband's tendency to wander. She gave them his photo, described his usual routes, and explained that he had dementia. That proactive step cut down the search time drastically the one night he did slip out. They found him within minutes, safe and sound.

THE ROLE OF TECHNOLOGY IN CAREGIVING

My First Encounter with "Smart" Solutions

About a decade ago, I visited a couple who had installed a home monitoring system. It tracked the mother's movements via motion sensors, sending alerts to the daughter's phone if something was amiss—like if Mom got up at 2 AM and didn't return to bed within a certain time frame. At first, I thought it might feel invasive. But the daughter said, "It's a lifesaver. I know when she's up and about. I can check on her before a small problem becomes a big one."

Available Technological Tools

- **Smart Home Devices**: Voice assistants like Amazon Echo or Google Home can remind about meds, appointments, or even to drink water. Smart locks can keep certain doors secured or allow you remote entry control.
- **Health Monitoring Apps**: Track vitals like blood pressure, heart rate, or even blood sugar if relevant. Some apps share data directly with physicians.
- **Remote Monitoring Systems**: Cameras or sensors that let you check in periodically. This is especially helpful if you can't be there 24/7.

Privacy & Ethical Considerations

This is a tricky topic. Dementia might reduce someone's capacity to fully consent, yet respecting their dignity is paramount.

- **Open Discussions**: Explain to your loved one, as best as possible, why you're using devices. Stress the goal: safety and well-being, not spying.

- **Balance**: Place cameras or sensors in high-risk zones, not in private areas like bathrooms.
- **Data Security**: Check how these devices store information. Make sure they have encryption or robust privacy settings.

I once knew a family who installed cameras in every room, including the bedroom. The mother felt violated, and her anxiety skyrocketed. Eventually, they realized they only needed cameras in communal areas and doorways, which restored her sense of privacy. Always consider how you'd feel in their shoes.

Benefits of Tech-Assisted Care

- **Efficiency**: Automatic pill dispensers ensure correct dosages at the right times.
- **Peace of Mind**: Remote monitoring means you don't have to guess if they're okay while you run an errand.
- **Reduced Stress**: Caregivers can catch small issues—like a missed meal—before they escalate.

One caretaker, Sandra, told me she used a simple app that alerted her if her father didn't open the fridge by noon. If he hadn't, she'd call to remind him to eat. It was subtle, noninvasive, and tremendously helpful in preventing him from skipping meals.

Selecting & Implementing Technology

- **Compatibility**: Does it work with your home's Wi-Fi or existing devices?
- **User-Friendliness**: Can your loved one, or you, operate it easily?
- **Trial Period**: If possible, test devices before fully committing. Some companies offer demos or free returns if it's not the right fit.

Remember, technology doesn't replace human connection. It complements your care. It can't replicate a warm smile or a gentle hand, but it can lift some burdens, giving you space to focus on what truly matters: quality time with your loved one.

PERSON-CENTERED CARE: CUSTOMIZING SPACES

The Heart of Personalization

In my early days, I met a sweet woman named Rose. She'd been an avid seamstress. Her sewing machine sat in the corner, though she rarely used it anymore. Her daughter decided to set up a small sewing nook, complete with fabrics and patterns Rose had loved. Even as Rose's skills faded, just being in that corner brought back warm memories of quilts she'd made over the years. She'd run her hand over the fabric, smile faintly, and say, "I used to stitch for hours, you know."

This is person-centered care in action: shaping the environment to reflect who they are, who they've been, and what they cherish.

Customizing Living Spaces

- **Photographs and Memorabilia**: A "memory wall" can do wonders. Arrange pictures from their youth, wedding, or children's milestones.
- **Favorite Colors & Themes**: If they loved the ocean, incorporate seashell motifs or shades of blue.
- **Soothing Elements**: Soft blankets, plush pillows, or a rocking chair that evokes memories of calm afternoons.

One man, Lionel, had a passion for jazz. His daughter painted music notes on one wall and kept a small speaker playing his favorite Ella Fitzgerald tunes. He'd hum along, content. Even if he forgot the lyrics, the rhythms were enough to soothe him.

Psychological Benefits of a Personalized Environment

Dementia can erode identity. Familiar surroundings can spark recollections, grounding them in a sense of self. A painting from a place they once visited, a trophy from a bowling league they once used to join—these items can stir fragments of memory. That spark of recognition can reduce agitation, brighten mood, and make day-to-day life feel less alien.

Examples of Successful Customization

- **Bedroom Transformation**: I recall a story of an older woman, Irene, who loved flowers. Her granddaughter helped decorate her room with floral curtains, bedding, and framed pictures of roses from Irene's own garden. Irene's mood lifted noticeably. She often pointed at the pictures, recalling the day she planted those roses.
- **Mini Home Museum**: Another family turned a hallway into a mini timeline of their father's life. Each section had photos from different decades: childhood, military service, wedding day, etc. He'd walk down that hallway, pausing at each set of photos, telling stories from his past to anyone who'd listen.

When environments resonate with a person's essence, daily confusion can ease. They feel recognized, validated, and less adrift in a fading memory.

LEVERAGING COMMUNITY FOR ENVIRONMENTAL SUPPORT

The Power of Community

During my years as a nurse, I've seen caregivers try to shoulder every burden alone. It's admirable but exhausting. Luckily, countless community resources exist to help make the home environment safer and more nurturing. Churches, non-profits, local senior centers—these can all be excellent places to seek help.

Local and National Support Options

- **Community Centers**: They often hold classes on home safety, memory training, or provide respite care. Check bulletin boards or local community websites for upcoming events.

- **Non-Profits**: Some organizations specialize in modifying homes for older adults or those with disabilities. They might install ramps, widen doorways, or provide grab bars free or at reduced cost.
- **Home Health Agencies**: Many offer occupational therapists who can evaluate your home, suggesting layout changes or safety modifications.

I recall a battered old van pulling up one day, carrying a team of volunteers from a local non-profit. They installed new lighting in the home of a patient who had dim, flickering bulbs. They added a second handrail on the stairwell. They even replaced the front step with a small ramp. The transformation was swift, and it cost the family nothing. I remember the patient's wife saying tearfully, "I can't believe strangers would do all this for us."

Benefits of Engaging Community Resources

- **Expert Advice**: Professionals who've seen it all can spot hazards you might overlook.
- **Support Networks**: Meeting other caregivers fosters a sense of camaraderie and shared understanding.
- **Social Interaction**: Some community activities are designed for dementia patients, like music therapy sessions or art classes.

When you attend these groups, you realize you're not alone. There's comfort in hearing someone else say, "I'm struggling with the same issue," and brainstorming solutions together.

Accessing Financial Aid or Grants

Home modifications can be pricey. Don't let that be a barrier. Investigate:

- **Government Programs**: Local or state agencies may provide grants for ramps, safety rails, or bathroom modifications.
- **Charitable Organizations**: The Alzheimer's Association, for instance, may guide you to funding resources.

- **Veterans Benefits**: If your loved one served in the military, they might qualify for assistance through the VA.

Research might be tedious, but the payoff is huge. One family I knew found a small grant that paid for a specialized bed and a new wheelchair ramp. It changed daily life for them, making transfers and movement much easier.

The Role of Community in Dementia Care

Collaboration is key. Talk to local businesses about becoming more dementia-friendly. Some grocery stores now offer "quiet hours," reducing noise and crowding for seniors with cognitive issues. Neighborhood watch programs can keep an eye out for neighbors who wander. There's so much potential when communities unite.

One inspiring example: a bakery in a small town started opening an hour early each week for seniors with dementia and their caregivers. The shop dimmed the lights, lowered the music, and set out large-print menus. People in the neighborhood said it quickly became a beloved social spot. Friendships formed over coffee and pastries. For many, it was the highlight of their week—a small slice of normalcy and kindness.

Pulling It All Together

Creating a dementia-friendly environment is not about making a home sterile or institutional. Quite the opposite. It's about adapting spaces so that your loved one is safe, comfortable, and gently guided through each day. That might mean installing door alarms or labeling cupboards. It might mean using voice assistants or big wall calendars. It definitely means injecting pieces of their personality into every corner—photos, mementos, familiar scents, or cherished music.

Remember, you're not in this alone. From local nonprofits to national helplines, from volunteer groups to new technology, help abounds if you know where to look. And every adjustment—no matter how minor—can lighten your burden and boost your loved one's sense of independence.

Picture yourself in six months, standing in a home that's been transformed. There are bright lights in the hall. A simple sign on the bathroom door. A bookshelf stocked with easy memory games. Maybe a monitored device that quietly reassures you your mom's still safe in bed. You notice less restlessness in her eyes, fewer anxious phone calls in the middle of the night. The two of you have found a new rhythm, a calmer routine.

Yes, dementia will still present hurdles. But your environment will no longer be one of them. With each step you take to reduce confusion or prevent accidents, you foster a space where the person you love can flourish in their own way. This is the goal of creating a dementia-friendly environment: to preserve dignity, reduce frustration, and keep the sense of "home" alive.

As we move forward to our next chapter, we'll explore communication and emotional connection—because, beyond physical spaces, the words we use and the empathy we convey matter just as much. For now, look around your living space. Think about what small tweak you can make today, and let that be the start of something bigger and brighter for you both.

COMMUNICATION AND EMOTIONAL CONNECTION

I never realized how powerful a single glance could be until I saw Mrs. Bates calm her husband with a gentle tilt of her head. He'd been pacing around the living room, lost in his own anxious world, muttering words that made little sense. She said nothing. She simply looked at him—soft eyes, a slight nod, and a tender press of her lips together—and he paused. His shoulders relaxed, and he moved closer to her like a moth to a comforting light. No words, just quiet understanding. If I hadn't witnessed it myself, I might not have believed how profoundly non-verbal communication can bridge gaps where dementia has severed so many verbal pathways.

In this chapter, we'll explore ways to connect with loved ones whose communication skills may be fading, morphing, or oscillating as dementia progresses. We'll delve into non-verbal cues, validation therapy, handling sundowning, deciphering emotional signals, and cultivating empathy. Finally, we'll circle back to why these connections matter so deeply—how they preserve relationships and affirm the humanity in every person, no matter how far they've drifted from our familiar world.

THE ART OF NON-VERBAL COMMUNICATION

When Words Fail, The Eyes Speak

Early in my nursing career, I cared for a retired teacher named Mr. Lawrence. He was known for his booming classroom voice. Yet, as dementia advanced, he retreated into near silence. His wife once confided, "He used to talk for hours about history or science. Now he just stares." It was heartbreaking. But one afternoon, I noticed something: whenever he was agitated, he'd grip the armrest of his wheelchair and turn his gaze toward the window. It was almost like he was asking for help, searching for a sign that he was safe. I started responding by gently placing my hand over his and leaning into his field of vision. That small gesture spoke volumes. His grip on the armrest eased, and he'd blink slowly, like a silent "thank you."

In dementia care, non-verbal communication often does the heavy lifting. Facial expressions can convey approval or anxiety in ways that words might never manage. Body language—like leaning forward, keeping arms uncrossed, and maintaining relaxed posture—tells your loved one, "I'm with you" or "I'm open to what you need." Eye contact can anchor someone who feels they're drifting, and a gentle smile can reassure them that they are not alone.

Practical Strategies for Non-Verbal Expression

- **Maintain Eye Contact**: Show that you're listening, that you see them. Even if their gaze wavers, consistently meeting their eyes can ground them.
- **Use Soft Touch**: A hand on the shoulder or a light stroke on the forearm can say, "I'm here," without speaking a single word. Of course, respect boundaries—if they recoil or stiffen, try another approach.
- **Vary Your Facial Expressions**: Don't be stoic. Smile warmly when you greet them, frown slightly if you sense their discomfort, and let concern show if they appear upset.

During one home visit, I saw a grandson quietly turn a subtle nod into a profound conversation with his grandmother. She'd raise an eyebrow, and he'd nod once, as if to say, "Yes, I understand." No spoken words were needed. In those gestures, they formed a dialogue.

Reading Their Non-Verbal Cues

Dementia can scramble language skills, but the body often broadcasts needs:

- **Restlessness or Fidgeting**: Could mean anxiety, boredom, or physical discomfort.
- **Avoiding Eye Contact**: Sometimes fear, sometimes overstimulation, or even embarrassment at not remembering something.
- **Furrowed Brows or Tight Lips**: Often signal frustration or confusion.

One of my patients, Ingrid, would purse her lips into a thin line whenever she needed to use the bathroom but didn't know how to articulate it. Recognizing that repetitive cue allowed her daughter to gently guide her before agitation escalated.

Building Non-Verbal Skills

Communication workshops or classes can help you sharpen these abilities. You might practice "mirroring" a partner's posture or facial expression, learning how subtle shifts can alter the emotional tone of an interaction. Observing how others respond to your own non-verbal signals can be enlightening. Are you inadvertently crossing your arms when frustrated? Are your shoulders tense, sending out nervous energy? By staying mindful, you can offer consistent, reassuring cues that your loved one can rely on.

I like to suggest to caregivers a daily "quiet check-in." For five minutes, sit with your loved one in silence. Watch their gestures, facial expressions, and breathing. Let them watch yours. Over time, you'll develop a shared language beyond words—one that gently says, "You matter. I'm here."

VALIDATION THERAPY TECHNIQUES: BUILDING TRUST

Stepping Into Their World

Validation therapy feels like a magic key sometimes. Instead of yanking someone back to "our" reality, you step into theirs. I recall Angela, a devout mother of three in her sixties, who was convinced her children were still toddlers. In her mind, they'd be returning from kindergarten any minute. She'd pace by the door, worried they might get lost on the way home. Her sister, exasperated, used to insist, "Your kids are grown! They're at work!" But that only upset Angela more. She'd stare, bewildered, tears pooling in her eyes.

Then we tried validation therapy. The sister gently said, "You miss them, don't you? You want to make sure they're safe." Angela nodded, relief washing over her face. With that acknowledgement, Angela's anxiety calmed. In time, she'd still ask, "When will they be back?" but the outbursts diminished. She felt heard. That's the essence of validation therapy— accepting the emotion beneath the confusion instead of dismissing it.

The Core Principles of Validation

- **1 Acknowledge Feelings**: Whether they're sad about a deceased parent or anxious over an imaginary appointment, honor the emotion first.
- **2 Avoid Correction and Confrontation**: Correcting only heightens tension. Gentle redirection or empathy fosters trust.
- **3 Enter Their Reality**: If they believe they're late for a meeting that doesn't exist, you might say, "That sounds important. Let's figure out how to help."

I once heard a caregiver respond to her mother's repeated claim that a stolen cat was in the house. Instead of saying, "Mom, that's impossible," she validated: "You must be worried about that cat. Let's see if we can find it and keep it safe." They never found a cat, of course, but her mother's agitation eased. Sometimes meeting someone in their perceived world is kinder than forcing them into yours.

Implementing Validation in Daily Life

- **Respond to the Emotion, Not the Fact**: If your father says, "I have to get to the office," he might be missing the purpose or routine work once provided. So you could respond, "You miss having important tasks, don't you?"
- **Use Reminiscing**: People with dementia often recall old memories more vividly than recent ones. Encouraging them to share stories about younger days can be soothing.
- **Stay Present & Patient**: This approach isn't about quick fixes. It's about building a sense of security over time.

Benefits for Both Caregiver and Patient

Validation therapy reduces conflict, plain and simple. When they feel understood, they resist less. They might cooperate more during daily tasks, like bathing or dressing. You, the caregiver, experience less stress because you're no longer trying to argue them into "reality." The relationship transforms from a battleground of correction to a place of mutual understanding. One caregiver told me, "It's like I finally got permission to stop fighting her delusions. Now I just let her guide me, and we find our way together."

SUNDOWNING: EVENING COMMUNICATION STRATEGIES

That Twilight Tension

Late afternoon shadows can bring more than just a darker sky. Many dementia patients grow restless, confused, or even aggressive as evening approaches—often called sundowning. I recall Mr. Chan, who'd spend all morning quietly enjoying his crossword puzzle but by 4 PM, he'd become irritable, snapping at his wife for seemingly no reason. She felt guilty, thinking she'd done something wrong. In truth, his brain was struggling to process the shift from daylight to dusk.

Why Sundowning Happens

The exact cause isn't fully understood, but routine disruptions, fatigue, or changes in lighting can all contribute. As darkness falls, people with dementia may misinterpret shadows or feel less secure. Biological clock confusion—circadian rhythms going awry—can also intensify agitation.

· · ·

Evening Communication Tactics

- **Soothing Rituals**: Establish a consistent early-evening routine, such as light snacks, soft music, or flipping through a photo album. Repetition cues the brain that it's time to wind down.
- **Environment Adjustments**: Keep the lights a bit brighter during twilight to minimize harsh shadows. Avoid loud TV shows or chaotic gatherings. A calm environment fosters calmer behavior.
- **Gentle Explanations**: If they're upset about not "finishing the day's work," you might say, "You've done so much today. Now it's time to relax." Offer reassurance, not arguments.

One caregiver told me she'd use a warm, lavender-scented hand massage for her mom each evening. She said the aroma seemed to ground her mother, reducing that restless energy. It was a small act, but powerful.

Handling Outbursts

When agitation flares, try to stay composed. If you speak in a panicked voice, they might mirror your distress. Use a soft tone, slow your words, and offer a calm presence. "I can see you're upset. I'm here with you," can be more effective than, "Stop it, calm down!" Also, allow extra time for them to process your words. Dementia can slow cognitive responses, so a brief pause can avert misunderstandings.

Remember: your patience can light up the dimming evening like a reassuring lantern. Even if they don't fully grasp your words, they'll sense your steady calm.

UNDERSTANDING AND INTERPRETING EMOTIONAL CUES

Emotions Unspoken

Sometimes, a distressed moan or repeated sigh can reveal more than a hundred words. Dementia can jumble language, but emotional signals often remain strong. I had a patient, Fiona, who'd furrow her brow and purse her lips whenever she needed a break from a noisy environment. If left in a crowded room too long, she'd start rocking slightly. Her family initially thought she was cold, draping a blanket over her shoulders, which only made her more agitated. Once they realized it was overstimulation, they'd move her to a quieter spot. Her face would relax almost immediately.

Practical Methods for Reading Emotions

- **Context Matters**: Where are they? Is it loud, bright, or chaotic? A meltdown might be triggered by environment, not necessarily anger or sadness.
- **Look for Clusters of Clues**: A single gesture can be ambiguous. But raised shoulders, tense hands, and a fixed stare altogether likely signal anxiety.
- **Ask Simple Questions**: If they can still speak a bit, gently ask, "Are you uncomfortable?" or "Is something bothering you?" Sometimes they'll confirm with a nod or a word.

Tailoring Your Response

Understanding emotional cues helps you respond effectively. If your loved one's body language screams discomfort, maybe it's time for a restroom break, a drink of water, or a change of scenery. If they seem anxious, a soothing approach—lowering your voice, offering gentle reassurance—can help them feel safe.

I once saw a daughter defuse her mother's growing agitation with a simple statement: "Mom, your face looks worried. Can I help?" Her mother hadn't spoken all day, but she exhaled and gave a slight nod. That moment of recognition was enough to break the cycle of tension.

Boosting Emotional Intelligence

Reflect daily on your loved one's moods and your reactions. Did a particular approach help? Or did it escalate things? Journaling can reveal patterns you might miss in the moment. You might notice, for instance, that morning confusion triggers restlessness, while after-lunch naps prevent afternoon crankiness. As you refine your awareness, you'll feel more confident anticipating their needs.

Also consider discussing concerns with a support group. Hearing others' stories often sparks new ideas: "Oh, that's how you handle it when your mom clenches her fists? I'll try that approach." Shared wisdom can expand your emotional toolkit exponentially.

EMPATHY IN ACTION: LISTENING AND RESPONDING

Why Empathy Transforms Care

Dementia isn't just about memory lapses; it's about navigating emotional terrain where fear, confusion, and frustration loom large. Empathy reminds your loved one that you're by their side. It says, "I see you, I feel for you, and I'll try to understand." This fosters trust—an invaluable commodity when someone's perception of reality keeps shifting.

I remember sitting with a man named Jacob, who had advanced dementia. He'd often babble about some distant memory—"The fish pond, we have to feed them!"—and get upset that no one else shared his concern. One day, I responded differently. I said, "That must feel urgent. Let's talk about the fish pond. What did you love about it?" His face lit up. He went on about lily pads and goldfish from decades ago. That empathetic listening changed everything. Instead of frustration, he found a willing ear, a safe space to reminisce.

Techniques for Active Listening

- **Reflect Emotions**: If they say, "I'm so worried," gently echo back: "You sound really anxious right now. Want to tell me more?"
- **Use Verbal Nods**: Simple interjections like "I see," "Oh," or "That's hard" keep the conversation flowing.
- **Lean In, Minimize Distractions**: Put down your phone, turn off the TV, and give them your full attention.

When your loved one sees that you're genuinely engaged, they're more likely to express themselves, even if it's in broken fragments.

Validating Feelings

Empathy often means avoiding statements like "Don't be silly" or "There's nothing to worry about." Instead, try: "I hear that you're worried. Let's figure this out." Even if their fear is irrational in our reality—like worrying about missing a bus at 10 PM—validate the emotion. "That bus ride seems important to you. Let's see how we can help you feel comfortable." This opens a door rather than slamming it shut.

Empathy Beyond Words

Empathy doesn't always require a verbal response. Sometimes it's a quiet presence, a hand squeeze, or a comforting hug. I've found that silence, accompanied by a gentle nod or a soft hum, can speak volumes. If your loved one is upset, just being there calmly can help them regulate their own emotions.

To hone this skill, consider role-playing with a friend or attending a local caregiver support group. Practice responding empathetically to hypothetical scenarios. It may feel awkward at first, but over time, empathy becomes second nature.

MAINTAINING RELATIONSHIPS AND EMOTIONAL BONDS

Why Bonds Matter

When we talk about relationships in the face of dementia, we're not just referencing the "good old days." We're acknowledging that even as memories fade, the emotional undercurrent between caregiver and patient can remain strong. That bond can buoy both of you through the roughest waters.

I recall the story of Tom and Lucy, married 51 years. Lucy's dementia had progressed to the point she rarely recognized Tom as her husband. Yet, whenever he hummed their wedding song, she'd rest her head on his shoulder, eyes closed in contentment. She might not have known the specifics— her name, the date, or the location of their wedding—but that gentle melody stirred an emotion deeper than memory.

Strategies for Nurturing Emotional Connections

- **Meaningful Activities**: Cook a favorite recipe together, watch old family videos, or take a walk in a garden that holds sentimental value. Shared experiences foster togetherness.
- **Family Involvement**: Encourage siblings, grandchildren, and close

friends to visit or call. Group gatherings, even if simple, keep social ties alive.

- **Celebrate Small Moments**: Did they smile when hearing an old lullaby? Did they giggle at a funny memory? Savor those glimpses of joy.

Overcoming Obstacles

Dementia can erode conversation skills, which can be disheartening. One day, your mom might chat cheerily about her childhood, and the next, she's silent or even hostile. Emotional distancing can occur, too. Perhaps your loved one withdraws because they're embarrassed about forgetting names or places.

I once knew a man who refused to attend family dinners because he couldn't keep track of who was who. He felt ashamed. The solution? The family started wearing name tags—really big ones with photos. It may sound silly, but it allowed him to re-engage without the pressure of perfect recall. Over time, that small adaptation rekindled connections he'd nearly lost.

The Payoff of Strong Bonds

When relationships stay strong, everyone benefits. Your loved one feels less alone, their quality of life improves, and they experience fewer bouts of anxiety. You, the caregiver, find renewed purpose and emotional satisfaction. One caregiver told me, "Every time she recognizes me, even for a moment, my heart soars. It's worth all the hard work."

Emotional bonds can also simplify day-to-day tasks. A patient who trusts you might be more willing to let you help with bathing or dressing. They might eat better or stay calmer because they sense the loving presence of someone who knows them beyond the disease. In these moments, you're reminded that beneath all the confusion, the person you love is still there, reaching out in ways big or small.

A Brief Reflection

Communication with someone who has dementia is never linear. It's a winding road of gestures, echoes of memories, and half-finished sentences. But it's also so much more. It's the reassuring touch of a hand, the validation of an emotion, the comforting routines that guide them through the unknown. It's understanding that when they're upset, it may be fear disguised as anger, or sadness cloaked in confusion. It's recognizing that love can outshine memory, that empathy can soothe the roughest day, and that a small nod or a gentle smile can mend a gap that words alone can't bridge.

Some days you might feel like you're failing—like no technique or therapy is making a dent. But remember, every interaction that carries understanding and patience is a victory. Every time you match your loved one's furrowed brow with a soft reassurance, you're weaving a thread of connection. Each moment of validation helps rebuild a trust that dementia tries to tear apart. Over time, these threads create a world of care—a testament that, despite a cruel disease, genuine communication is still possible.

So let your face speak volumes when words slip away. Let your empathy gently cradle their anxieties. And cherish every flicker of recognition, every hint of joy, every quiet comfort that passes between you. Because in the realm of dementia, these fleeting bonds aren't small or insignificant. They're everything.

Practical Takeaways & Exercises

- **Non-Verbal Check-In**: Spend five minutes in silence each day, observing your loved one's facial expressions and gestures. Practice mirroring or responding with your own calm demeanor.
- **Validation Practice**: When they mention something that seems "unreal," respond to the emotion behind it. If they're scared of missing an event, acknowledge that fear rather than dismissing it.
- **Sundowning Journal**: Keep notes on what happens during late afternoon or evening. Note lighting, noise, activities. Over time, see if patterns emerge that help you adjust the routine.
- **Emotional Cue Index**: Make a quick reference list of your loved one's common body language signs—like a clenched fist for anxiety or tapping fingers for boredom. Refer to it when they exhibit those signals.
- **Empathy Role-Play**: With a friend or family member, simulate a brief scenario where one person is confused or upset, and the other

responds with validation and empathy. Discuss afterward what worked or felt comforting.

- **Relationship Reflection**: Once a week, recall a moment when you truly connected with your loved one—maybe a shared laugh or a tender silence. Write it down. Remembering these moments fuels resilience.

In the next chapter, we'll explore the daily challenges caregivers face—those seemingly endless tasks and obstacles that test patience and stamina. We'll talk practical solutions, building on the communication techniques from this chapter to ensure your caregiving approach remains holistic and grounded in empathy. Because at the end of the day, being heard and understood—whether by word, gesture, or gentle touch—is at the heart of every meaningful connection. And in dementia care, that connection is what keeps both your spirits afloat.

DAILY CAREGIVING CHALLENGES
AND SOLUTIONS

I remember walking into Mrs. Dwyer's living room one bright morning. She was gently helping her husband, Harold, put on a pair of slippers. He fumbled with the heel for a few seconds, then paused. I could see the confusion clouding his face—like he wasn't quite sure where his foot ended and the slipper began. Mrs. Dwyer rested a hand on his knee, smiled, and calmly said, "It's okay. Let's do this step by step." In that simple phrase, she captured so much of what daily caregiving is about: patience, empathy, and a willingness to adapt the ordinary. This chapter is all about those moments—about taking challenges that once felt daunting and breaking them down into manageable, caring acts.

We've spent previous chapters exploring the foundations of dementia, the environment we create at home, and the importance of clear communication. Now, we move into the heart of everyday life: those tasks and routines that fill the day from sunrise to bedtime. You'll learn how to simplify activities of daily living (ADLs), manage aggression when it flares up, plan nutritious meals, organize medications, encourage meaningful engagement, and troubleshoot sleep issues. Because, as we've seen throughout this journey, caregiving isn't just about big revelations. It's about the small, daily triumphs that remind both you and your loved one: there is still joy, purpose, and dignity in each moment spent together.

ADLS: SIMPLIFYING DAILY TASKS

The Cornerstones of Independence

ADLs stand for "Activities of Daily Living," and they form the backbone of our everyday existence. Getting dressed, brushing teeth, taking a shower, preparing a simple meal—these are tasks we often do on autopilot. Dementia, however, interrupts that autopilot and replaces it with uncertainty. I saw this with a former patient, Mr. Jones, who would stand in front of his closet, staring at his shirts for several minutes, unable to decide which one to wear or how to put it on. He felt embarrassed, as though he'd lost a piece of himself. That's the power of ADLs. When someone struggles with them, they can feel as if their independence is slipping away.

Basic ADLs (bathing, dressing, feeding) are essential for personal care. Instrumental ADLs (cooking, cleaning, shopping) are more complex, involving planning and decision-making. When these become difficult, caregivers need to step in. But stepping in doesn't mean taking over entirely. On the contrary, one of the most crucial strategies is to find ways to let your loved one participate as much as they can. It could be as simple as choosing which shirt to wear or picking which cereal to eat for breakfast. These small choices can preserve dignity and reinforce a sense of control.

Breaking Tasks into Manageable Steps

One morning, as I was helping a woman named Pilar, she became frustrated while trying to brush her hair. She kept tangling the brush in the same spot. Instead of brushing for her, I gently guided her hand, saying, "Let's do the top first. Now the sides." We took a moment to celebrate when she got through one section without getting stuck. Gradually, her frown turned into a small smile. This is the essence of "task segmentation"—dividing a task into clear, simple steps, and allowing your loved one to focus on one mini-goal at a time.

- **Focus on One Action at a Time**: "Pick up your shirt," then "Place your arm through the sleeve."
- **Use Adaptive Equipment**: Velcro shoes instead of laces, slip-on pants with elastic waistbands, or a shower seat for extra support.
- **Keep Praise Flowing**: Even a small success matters. "You did great picking the outfit today."

The Power of Routine and Lists

Routines anchor us in familiarity, especially in the midst of dementia. Creating a consistent schedule—waking up, brushing teeth, getting dressed, having breakfast—reduces confusion and shortens the time spent wondering, "What do I do next?" I once worked with a family who wrote out a morning checklist. They pinned it to the fridge, with photos illustrating each step: a toothbrush, a shirt, a cereal bowl, etc. Every time Grandpa Frank completed one item, he'd check it off. It became a small ceremony of accomplishment.

- **Morning & Evening Rituals**: Repetition helps memory retention.
- **Task Tracking**: A bulletin board or a laminated list can guide daily chores.
- **Encourage Participation**: Let them cross off completed tasks or place a sticker next to them.

Having a routine doesn't mean life becomes rigid. It simply lays down a comforting blueprint that can be adapted if needed. That sense of predictability can ease anxiety for both caregiver and patient, allowing you to focus on enjoying the day rather than putting out fires at every turn.

Fostering Autonomy and Choice

Dementia may affect memory or coordination, but it doesn't erase the need for independence. Where possible, offer your loved one choices. Maybe they can pick between two outfits or decide whether to have toast or oatmeal for breakfast. Even small decisions can bolster self-esteem. I recall Linda, a caregiver who told her mom, "You can choose which shoes to wear—these red ones or these blue ones." Her mother, who rarely spoke, pointed to the blue pair and beamed as Linda helped her slip them on.

Keep in mind that autonomy doesn't mean leaving them to struggle alone. It's a balancing act: stepping in when needed, stepping back when they can manage on their own. It's about guiding rather than controlling, encouraging rather than demanding. And it's about celebrating every tiny victory, from buttoning a shirt to lifting a spoon. Because in these small moments, your loved one reclaims a piece of themselves.

HANDLING AGGRESSION AND AGITATION

Seeing the Person Behind the Anger

Aggression can blindside you. One minute your father is calm; the next, he's red-faced and yelling at you for "moving his keys" or "throwing out his favorite hat." It's jarring, especially when it comes from someone who used to be gentle and kind. But in my years working with dementia patients, I've learned that aggression or agitation is almost always a symptom, not a personality shift. It often signals discomfort, confusion, or fear that they can't fully articulate.

Take Marilyn's husband, George. He'd fly into a rage whenever the TV was on too loud. They eventually realized he wasn't really angry at Marilyn —he was overwhelmed by the noise. Once they lowered the volume or turned it off entirely, he calmed. That's the key: figure out what's sparking the outburst, and address that root cause.

Recognizing Triggers and Early Warnings

- **Environmental Stressors**: Loud music, cluttered rooms, crowded gatherings, or glaring lights can overload the senses.
- **Routine Changes**: A missed nap, a delayed meal, or an unexpected visitor may unsettle them.
- **Physical Discomfort**: Pain, thirst, needing to use the bathroom— these can turn into agitation if unmet.

Sometimes you'll notice early warning signs—like fidgeting hands, pacing, or raised voices. If you spot these signals, intervene gently. Maybe it's time for a quieter space, a glass of water, or a comforting hand on their shoulder.

De-Escalation Techniques

- **Stay Composed**: Keep your tone calm and your voice low. If your stress level spikes, they'll likely mirror it.

- **Offer Distraction**: "Hey, let's go look at that photo album," or "Would you like some tea?" Shifting focus can break the cycle of escalation.
- **Use Reassuring Language**: "I see you're upset. I want to help you feel better." This acknowledges their emotion without arguing about facts.

I recall one especially tense moment with Mr. Ortega, who would repeatedly accuse his daughter of hiding his favorite newspaper. She discovered that placing an old stack of local papers on the coffee table soothed him. He'd find "his" paper whenever he wanted it, and the accusations vanished. A small tweak, but it changed their entire day-to-day dynamic.

Crafting a Calming Environment

There's a reason spas are designed with soft lighting, gentle music, and minimal clutter: calm surroundings invite calm feelings. For dementia patients, this approach can be invaluable:

- **Dim Overhead Lights** and rely on lamps or natural light.
- **Declutter** to reduce visual chaos.
- **Soothing Sounds**: Instrumental music, nature sounds, or even a light windchime can help.

Try a scented candle or aromatherapy if they find it comforting, but keep safety in mind. Also consider your own stress. During an outburst, take a few slow, deep breaths. Count to five on each inhale, hold for a moment, then exhale. That short pause can help you respond rather than react.

Caregiver Self-Care During Incidents

It's tough not to take aggression personally, especially if cruel words are being hurled in your direction. But remind yourself: it's the disease talking. Step out of the room if you need to regroup. Ask a family member or neighbor for help, or use respite care resources if outbursts become frequent. You can't pour from an empty cup. Keeping your emotional balance will help you come back with empathy instead of frustration.

One caregiver, Sam, told me how he'd learned to do a quick visualization exercise whenever his father lashed out. He'd picture himself stepping into a calm, blue ocean, letting the waves wash away his anger. It might sound whimsical, but for Sam, it was a mental reset. He'd return with a gentle tone, say, "Dad, I'm here for you," and it usually made a difference.

MEAL PLANNING AND NUTRITION FOR DEMENTIA PATIENTS

Fuel for Body and Mind

Sitting down to a meal might seem straightforward, but for someone with dementia, it can be a confusing process. Which fork do I use? Is this my plate? Did I already eat breakfast? Nutritional needs also change. Some patients lose their appetite; others forget to drink water and risk dehydration. Balanced meals matter not just for physical health but also for cognitive function. A good diet can help stabilize mood, energy, and possibly slow mental decline.

Simplifying Meal Prep

I once visited Ms. Beatriz, who adored cooking but found it stressful to manage big meals. We turned her kitchen into a more dementia-friendly space. Ingredients were labeled and pre-portioned. We used color-coded measuring cups, and we stuck to simple, hearty recipes—like vegetable soup or baked chicken with carrots. She felt proud she could still "cook for the family" with minimal risk or confusion.

- **Easy-to-Prepare Dishes**: Soups, casseroles, and slow-cooker recipes often require fewer steps.
- **Incorporate Favorites**: Familiar flavors can awaken appetite and memories.
- **Encourage Participation**: Let them chop softer veggies or stir batter if it's safe.

Overcoming Eating Difficulties

- **Modify Textures**: Cut food into bite-sized pieces, or even blend or puree if swallowing is an issue.
- **Create a Calm Dining Environment**: Lower background noise, provide good lighting, and avoid visual clutter on the table.

- **Use Contrasting Plates**: A white plate on a light tablecloth might be hard to see. Bright plate colors make the food more distinct.

Some families find that finger foods—like small sandwich squares, vegetable sticks, or fruit slices—help maintain independence in eating. Also, consider how hydration can slip: offer water frequently, maybe with a squeeze of lemon or a few cucumber slices for flavor.

Keeping it Appealing and Fun

Making meals a positive event can spark interest. Put on soft music, set the table nicely, or arrange food in a colorful way. Sometimes, I've seen caregivers incorporate "theme nights"—like a mini "Italian dinner" with a simple pasta dish and red-checkered napkins. Even if it's a small detail, it can bring enjoyment, turning a mundane meal into a mini celebration.

Don't forget snacks if big meals feel overwhelming. Sometimes, small frequent bites throughout the day work better than sitting down for three large meals. The goal isn't to be fancy or elaborate; it's to ensure consistent, nutritious intake that keeps your loved one energized and engaged.

MEDICATION MANAGEMENT: BEST PRACTICES

The Weight of a Tiny Pill

It's astonishing how something so small—like a pill—can carry such importance. Dementia often comes with a range of prescriptions: some for cognitive support, some for mood regulation, others for physical health. Juggling them all can be stressful. One missed dose might lead to confusion; doubling up accidentally can be dangerous. In my early days, I met a lovely woman who meticulously sorted her husband's pills into color-coded boxes each Sunday. She'd say, "It's my weekly puzzle, but at least I know he's safe."

Organizing and Scheduling

- **Pill Boxes**: Simple, cheap, and effective. Some have compartments for morning, noon, evening, and bedtime.

- **Digital Alarms**: Set reminders on your phone or a dedicated medication app. The alarm rings when it's time to administer meds.
- **Written Schedules**: A chart that lists each medication, dosage, and time can clarify confusion if multiple family members help with care.

I often recommend the "Medisafe" app to families as it has a feature that requires taking a photo of the caregiver giving the pill. Some find it a bit high-tech, but it gives them peace of mind, especially when different home aides rotate shifts. They can see in real-time that their loved one's midday pill has been taken.

Administering Medications Wisely

Sometimes, it's not just about remembering to give the pill. It's how to administer it:

- **Crushing Pills**: Only if the doctor or pharmacist says it's okay. Some meds shouldn't be crushed.
- **Hiding in Food**: A spoonful of applesauce or yogurt can help if swallowing is an issue.
- **Establish a Routine**: Tie medication times to daily rituals, like breakfast or bedtime routines.

Be mindful of side effects. If you notice unusual drowsiness, agitation, or changes in appetite soon after starting a new medication, report it. Your loved one might need a dosage adjustment or a different prescription altogether. Regular check-ins with the doctor keep the regimen optimized.

Regular Reviews and Adjustments

Dementia is progressive, and so are its medication needs. Periodic reviews with a healthcare provider help ensure each drug is still beneficial. Possibly they need a new medication for anxiety or to taper off something no longer effective. Keep notes on any changes—did they sleep better after the dose was reduced? Did aggression decrease when the timing changed? Sharing these observations can guide the doctor to refine the plan.

Medication management can feel like a second job, but once you establish a system, it becomes part of the daily rhythm. And remember: you don't have to figure it out alone. Pharmacists can explain drug interactions, doctors can adjust prescriptions, and technology can keep you on track. That synergy can transform medication chaos into a reassuring routine.

ENCOURAGING ACTIVITY AND ENGAGEMENT

The Spark of Participation

Even with memory hiccups, a person's innate passions can linger. Think of a dad who used to love fixing cars or a grandma who sang in the church choir. Dementia doesn't erase those interests; it just means we might have to adapt them. One day, I watched a caregiver lead her mother in a gentle stretching routine. Her mother used to be a dance instructor, so she added soft music, gave her mother a "ballet bar" (it was really just a sturdy chair), and they did slow, graceful movements together. Her mother's face lit up. Movement tapped into muscle memory and spirit, giving her a sense of purpose.

Physical and Cognitive Activities

- **Arts and Crafts**: Painting, coloring books, knitting, or collages can engage creativity and fine motor skills.
- **Gentle Exercises**: Short walks in the backyard, chair yoga, or stationary cycling. A bit of movement can lift mood and help with circulation.
- **Puzzles & Games**: Simple crosswords, large-piece jigsaw puzzles, or word matching can keep the brain active. Adjust the difficulty level so it's challenging but not frustrating.

I once worked with a man who had been an avid chess player. His wife adapted the game by removing some pieces, simplifying the board to just a few pawns and the king. He played "mini-chess," and while it wasn't exactly the grand matches he once enjoyed, it still sparked excitement in him. He'd proudly exclaim, "Check!" even if it wasn't quite accurate. That didn't matter. The joy was real.

The Social Dimension

Isolation can worsen confusion and depression. Planning occasional social engagements—even small ones—helps break monotony. Invite neighbors for tea, or arrange a short visit with grandchildren. If large crowds overwhelm your loved one, keep gatherings small. Or consider community centers that offer dementia-friendly classes or music therapy sessions. Shared laughter, casual conversation, and the warmth of others can provide a sense of belonging that's crucial for mental health.

Encourage family and friends to participate in these activities, too. Maybe a niece helps with painting or a grandson joins a simple cooking session. These interactions remind everyone that the person with dementia is still very much alive inside, with stories to share and moments to create.

Adapting and Personalizing

Always tailor activities to personal history and abilities. If your mother once baked elaborate cakes, let her do simpler tasks like stirring batter or decorating cookies. If your father loved the outdoors, set up a small indoor garden or a windowsill herb kit. The key is to keep the spirit of the activity intact while adjusting for current limitations. And don't be afraid to pivot if something isn't working. Flexibility is your friend in dementia care. What matters most is engagement, not perfection.

Lastly, savor these moments of connection. They can be fleeting, but they hold such richness. Whenever I joined an activity with a patient, I'd often leave feeling unexpectedly uplifted. Because in these shared experiences—no matter how small—there's a reminder that hope and joy can coexist with dementia. A quiet victory, a simple creation, or a shared laugh can outshine many of the day's frustrations.

SOLUTIONS FOR SLEEP DISTURBANCES

Why Sleep Matters So Much

A good night's sleep can shape the entire next day—mood, energy, and cognitive clarity hinge on restful slumber. In dementia, however, sleep often becomes fragmented. Some patients wake multiple times a night, confused and restless. Others experience sundowning, where they grow agitated just as evening sets in. Insomnia, nightmares, or nighttime wandering can leave both caregiver and patient utterly drained.

I recall Ms. Garrett, whose husband, Larry, would pace the hallway at 2 AM, convinced he needed to "go to work." She tried reasoning with him, which only fueled his agitation. Together, we crafted a soothing bedtime routine—soft lights, calming music, a mug of warm milk, and a reassurance that his "work" was done for the day. It didn't fix everything overnight, but he started sleeping more deeply and waking less.

Creating a Sleep-Friendly Environment

- **Consistent Bedtime Ritual**: Like a bedtime story for kids, grown-ups with dementia benefit from a predictable wind-down—maybe a gentle hand massage or reading a short passage from a familiar book.
- **Control Lighting**: Ensure the bedroom is dark enough for rest, but use a small nightlight if total darkness triggers fear.
- **Temperature & Comfort**: A slightly cooler room often promotes better sleep. Make sure bedding is cozy but not too heavy.

Encourage daytime activities (physical or social) so they feel pleasantly tired by evening. But avoid big naps late in the afternoon, which might jumble the body's internal clock. A short midday rest is fine, but four hours of napping can lead to midnight restlessness.

Addressing Nighttime Wandering

If they get up in the middle of the night, gently guide them back to bed, reassure them they're safe, and dim the lights. Some caregivers find motion sensors helpful—if a loved one leaves the bedroom, they receive an alert, allowing them to intervene before the wandering escalates. In extreme cases, it might be necessary to secure doors or place alarms to ensure safety. The key is to maintain dignity while preventing risk.

Monitoring and Seeking Help

Keep a sleep diary. Note what time they go to bed, how often they wake, and any triggers like caffeine or a late meal. If chronic insomnia or severe sundowning persists, consult a healthcare professional. There might be underlying medical issues like sleep apnea or restless leg syndrome. Or medication side effects could be interfering with rest. Doctors can sometimes adjust prescriptions or suggest melatonin or other sleep aids, though these require careful supervision.

A good night's rest isn't a luxury—it's foundational. Both you and your loved one deserve to greet each day with as much energy and clarity as possible. While no single strategy works for everyone, a combination of routine, environment, and gentle reassurance can significantly improve the odds of a peaceful night.

A Brief Wrap-Up and a Look Ahead

Dementia reshapes our approach to basic tasks. It challenges our patience and creativity. But as we've discovered, there's a wealth of strategies for tackling daily caregiving hurdles. From simplifying ADLs to managing aggression, from planning meals to ensuring restful sleep, each tip is like a small piece of a larger tapestry—a tapestry that, when woven together, forms a compassionate, supportive environment for your loved one.

Yes, the day-to-day can feel overwhelming. Tying shoes, calming an outburst, dishing up balanced meals, juggling pill schedules, organizing engaging activities, and hoping everyone sleeps well—these tasks add up. But in each of these duties lies an opportunity: an opportunity to connect, to nurture independence, and to show unwavering care.

You don't walk this path alone. Remember the supportive networks you've encountered: friends, family, local groups, healthcare professionals. Rely on them. Share your victories and your struggles. Even the smallest triumph—like seeing your loved one smile after successfully putting on a sweater—can fuel you for the next challenge.

In our upcoming chapter, we'll delve deeper into legal, financial, and ethical considerations. Because while the day-to-day is crucial, so is preparing for the future, ensuring that you have the proper documents, plans, and protections in place. It might not be as hands-on as feeding or bathing, but it's every bit as important for safeguarding your loved one's well-being.

For now, though, take a moment to acknowledge how far you've come. You've learned to adapt, to empathize, to break tasks into smaller steps, and to find the beauty in everyday routines. Those glimpses of patience and understanding you offer each day aren't just solutions; they're gifts—gifts of dignity, hope, and love that resonate far beyond the present moment. And that's what truly matters on this caregiving journey.

LEGAL, FINANCIAL, AND ETHICAL CONSIDERATIONS

⚜

When I first met Margaret, she was clutching a worn binder labeled "Important Papers." Its edges were frayed, like it had been flipped through a thousand times. She walked me to the small kitchen table, breathing deeply as she set the binder down. Inside were documents—some dated a decade ago, some brand-new. She tapped the stack and said, "I'm terrified of messing up. He always handled everything, and now... now it's on me." Her husband, George, had advanced dementia. He could no longer make sense of numbers or even recall their home address. Margaret felt overwhelmed. But she also felt a fierce responsibility to protect the life they'd built. This chapter is about that feeling—about stepping into a labyrinth of legal forms, financial decisions, and ethical puzzles, all while caring for someone whose mind is slipping away. You're not alone. Let's find a path together.

We've explored the day-to-day challenges of caregiving, from communication hurdles to ensuring safe, meaningful routines. Yet beneath those daily tasks looms a series of vital questions: Who will speak for your loved one when they cannot speak for themselves? How do you finance prolonged care without losing the family home? What happens when medical interventions clash with personal beliefs or your loved one's earlier wishes? These legal, financial, and ethical concerns might feel daunting. But trust me—I've seen caregivers navigate them successfully by arming themselves with knowledge, empathy, and a willingness to plan ahead. Let's delve into the tools, documents, and principles that will help you protect your loved one's dignity and your own peace of mind.

UNDERSTANDING POWER OF ATTORNEY

Stepping Into Their Shoes

Years ago, I cared for a retired mechanic named Vince. He was a meticulous man, with blackened nails and a brain that once hummed with mechanical logic. After dementia took hold, he forgot how to pay bills or withdraw money for groceries. His daughter, Amanda, realized they needed a legal mechanism to help manage his finances. That's when she discovered Power of Attorney (POA). She once told me, "I'm not trying to control his life. I just want to ensure he's safe and his bills get paid." That's the heart of POA: stepping into someone's shoes, not to dominate them, but to safeguard their well-being and finances.

Power of Attorney is a legal document granting one person (the agent) authority to act on behalf of another (the principal). This can include handling money, signing checks, or making medical decisions—depending on the type of POA. There's a general POA, which gives broad powers, and a durable POA, which remains valid even if the principal becomes mentally incapacitated. A healthcare POA (or medical POA) focuses specifically on healthcare decisions. All these versions exist to fill a crucial gap: What happens when your loved one can no longer make decisions independently?

The Process and the Responsibilities

Acquiring a POA typically involves filling out state-specific forms and having them notarized. You ought to get a lawyer's guidance when getting a POA. They'll clarify which POA suits your situation and ensure all legal boxes are checked. One family I supported actually found free legal clinics that helped them finalize the documents.

But remember: with authority comes accountability. If you have a financial POA, you can manage bank accounts, sell property, or even adjust investments on your loved one's behalf. However, you can't typically alter their will or vote for them. If you only have a financial POA, you can't make healthcare calls—unless you also have a medical POA. Acting in the best interest of the principal is paramount. When Amanda took over Vince's finances, she kept careful logs. She told me, "It felt like I was stepping into Dad's workshop, making sure every tool stayed in its place."

Selecting the right agent matters. They should be trustworthy, organized, and willing to shoulder emotional burdens. Sometimes that's you—the primary caregiver. Sometimes it's another relative or even a professional. Think about reliability, availability, and the capacity to remain calm under stress. If your loved one can express a preference, respect it. If not, consider who best aligns with their values. POA is a weighty but vital shield, protecting them when life's storms come knocking.

ADVANCED DIRECTIVES AND THEIR IMPORTANCE

Safeguarding Their Voice

I recall a heartbreaking scene: A woman named Louisa stood in a hospital hallway, tears in her eyes, being asked if her mother would want a feeding tube. Her mother couldn't speak anymore. Louisa didn't know. Nobody had talked about it beforehand. She whispered, "How do I decide something this big?" Advanced directives exist to spare you that agony. They serve as your loved one's voice when their own voice has faded.

Advanced directives are legal documents dictating medical wishes if a person becomes unable to communicate. A living will spells out desired (or undesired) treatments, such as ventilators, resuscitation, or feeding tubes. A healthcare proxy or healthcare POA appoints someone to make medical decisions, guided by known preferences. Imagine them as a roadmap left behind, so you're not making blind guesses in emotionally charged moments.

The Creation and the Peace of Mind

Drafting advanced directives involves frank conversations. Ask your loved one about end-of-life care, comfort measures, or potential interventions. Doctors can clarify the medical ramifications of different choices. A lawyer can outline your state's specific requirements—some states mandate witnesses or notaries. Once signed, keep copies handy. Share them with close family, the appointed proxy, and relevant healthcare providers.

Having these directives brings a unique calm. Family arguments about "what Mom would've wanted" diminish when her wishes are in writing. If your loved one strongly opposes life support or insists on it, that clarity can guide doctors. It's not about being morbid. It's about preserving dignity. Sandra, a caregiver I knew, said it best: "Mom's living will felt like a comforting anchor. Even though she wasn't well enough to speak, she was still steering her own ship."

Obstacles may surface. Some relatives might resist, hoping to prolong life at any cost. Others might struggle with cultural or religious concerns. Approach these conflicts with patience. Emphasize that advanced directives honor the patient's autonomy. If disagreements persist, consider a mediator or a family meeting with medical staff. The goal is to ensure your loved one's values remain front and center, even in their silence.

FINANCIAL PLANNING FOR LONG-TERM CARE

Counting the True Cost

The first time I heard a caregiver mention "we might lose the house," my heart sank. Dementia care can be financially draining. In-home help, adult day programs, assisted living facilities, skilled nursing care—each option comes with a price. The unpredictability of disease progression means you might need more resources than you initially thought. This is why planning early is crucial. One family I knew actually sat down with a financial advisor as soon as their dad was diagnosed. They said, "We wanted no surprises. We wanted to keep Dad comfortable without bankrupting ourselves."

Think about the cost of in-home care if you choose that route. You might pay hourly for a home health aide, or possibly 24/7 care. Factor in modifications like wheelchair ramps or bathroom supports. If facility-based care is needed, monthly fees can be substantial, especially for specialized memory care units. Start by mapping out a comprehensive budget. Tally everything from medical visits to grocery bills to the possibility of respite care. Then consider what financial assistance might be available.

Exploring Assistance and Savings

Some caregivers rely on Medicaid, which can cover long-term care if income and assets meet eligibility criteria. Others look into Medicare, though it's more limited for long-term coverage. Non-profits sometimes offer grants or sliding-scale services. A longtime caregiver I worked with last year discovered a local nonprofit that provided short respite stays for free. "I genuinely felt like I'd stumbled on a hidden treasure," he said, relieved.

Long-term care insurance is another option. It can offset expenses for home care, assisted living, or skilled nursing. But policies vary widely. Some only kick in after a certain waiting period, others might exclude pre-existing conditions. If you or your loved one have a policy, read the fine print. Additionally, consider a special needs trust. It safeguards assets for someone with a disability (including advanced dementia) without compromising Medicaid eligibility. Usually, an attorney's guidance is helpful here.

When funds are tight, prioritize essential expenses: food, medications, safe shelter. Speak openly with family about the possibility of pooling resources. Some communities have volunteer programs or local seniors' groups that provide free or low-cost assistance. As the Jeffersons said, "We realized we didn't have to do it all alone. There were more pockets of help out there than we ever imagined."

NAVIGATING INSURANCE AND BENEFITS

Insurance as a Lifeline—But Read the Fine Print

Insurance can be a godsend when facing the steep costs of dementia care. Yet, policies can feel like a labyrinth of clauses and disclaimers. I recall helping an older couple decipher their policy. They discovered it didn't cover the memory care program they were counting on. They felt betrayed. That's why it's crucial to thoroughly understand health insurance coverage, including co-pays, deductibles, and exclusions. If you have long-term care insurance, verify what triggers coverage—some require the inability to perform specific ADLs before they pay out.

Filing claims can be tedious. Keep meticulous records: doctor's notes, receipts for medical equipment, proof of in-home care hours. A friend of mine, whose mother had dementia, kept a binder with all relevant paperwork. She'd note every phone call with the insurance rep, including date and time. "It saved my sanity," she confided. Whenever a dispute arose, she had facts at her fingertips.

Government Programs and Overcoming Denials

For those with limited income, Medicaid can cover significant portions of long-term care. Eligibility rules vary by state, so it's wise to consult with a benefits counselor or attorney. Medicare might cover short rehabilitative stays or hospice services, but not prolonged custodial care. Meanwhile,

Supplemental Security Income (SSI) can provide monthly financial aid if your resources are low.

Insurance denials happen. Sometimes a claim is labeled "not medically necessary," or you get stuck in red tape. Don't lose heart. Gather your documents, politely but firmly appeal. If needed, a social worker or attorney can help you challenge a denial. Some caregivers also contact local government representatives if they sense unfair treatment. It might sound drastic, but I've seen letter-writing campaigns magically open bureaucratic doors. The key is persistence. Remember, insurance is supposed to help your loved one get needed care—not become an obstacle.

ETHICAL DILEMMAS IN DEMENTIA CARE

Balancing Safety and Autonomy

One day, I visited a sweet gentleman named Henry who insisted on going for solo walks around his block. He was unsteady, disoriented, and occasionally forgot his address. His wife, Rosa, was frantic, afraid he'd wander off and get lost. But Henry felt caged if she forbid him to go. This tug-of-war— ensuring someone's safety while honoring their independence—is a prime ethical challenge. Dementia shifts the balance of power. You might have to say "no" for their own good, but how do you do it without eroding their dignity?

Autonomy says respect their choices. Beneficence says protect them from harm. These principles collide often in dementia care. Another ethical dilemma might involve end-of-life decisions. Should we continue aggressive treatments if your loved one is in advanced stages, or focus on comfort? If they never expressed a preference, you're left guessing. This guesswork can strain families, especially if siblings disagree.

Finding Guidance and Resolution

Open communication helps. Arrange family meetings with all key parties. Present the facts, discuss the person's prior stated values if known, and see if you can find common ground. Sometimes, a care team meeting with doctors, social workers, or an ethics committee can clarify best steps. I recall a family who engaged a hospital ethics committee when deciding whether to insert a feeding tube. Each member brought heartfelt concerns.

Hearing them validated and weighed by professionals helped them unify on a course of action that felt morally right.

You might also face moral quandaries around using "therapeutic fibs." For instance, telling your loved one a small untruth to prevent distress. Is that manipulative or humane? In practice, many caregivers decide that if it spares undue agony, a gentle redirection or white lie can be kinder than forcing them to confront a painful truth repeatedly. The line can blur, so rely on your own moral compass and possibly a professional counselor's input. Remember, no single rulebook covers all dementia care scenarios. Ethical caregiving thrives on empathy, reflection, and the courage to adjust when needed.

PROACTIVE STRATEGIES FOR FUTURE CARE NEEDS

Planning Is a Gift to Everyone

If there's one message I could shout from the rooftops, it's this: planning early gives you a priceless head start. Dementia is progressive, and changes may come faster than you expect. I once knew a nurse who discovered, almost overnight, that her mother needed round-the-clock care. She told me, "I wish we'd discussed this before it became a crisis." That's the essence of proactive planning. It spares you from scrambling in emergencies, letting you calmly map out possible paths.

Start by assessing your loved one's current stage and probable future needs. Will in-home care suffice for the foreseeable future? If not, are you open to a memory care facility? Are you financially and emotionally prepared for the cost and transition? By anticipating these questions, you can make informed moves. You might, for instance, convert a ground-floor room into a bedroom if stairs become unmanageable. Or discuss with siblings how you'll share responsibilities. Regularly revisit these plans, because dementia rarely follows a neat timeline.

Building a Long-Term Care Roadmap

Financial preparedness is a cornerstone. As we've covered, this might involve insurance, savings, or exploring government benefits. But it's also emotional readiness—understanding that your loved one might eventually forget your name, become bedridden, or need hospice. It's tough to face, but it's kinder in the long run. When the moment arrives, you'll already have a blueprint.

Care planning guides and financial planning software can be lifesavers. They prompt you to list assets, estimate costs, and set up a timeline for major decisions. Think of them as checklists for the future. They won't solve every problem, but they'll keep you from overlooking crucial details. Stay flexible. If your loved one's condition worsens unexpectedly, you may need to accelerate certain steps. That's okay. Adjust, pivot, and keep communication open with family and professionals.

Finally, remember that proactive planning is an act of love. It reduces last-minute chaos and ensures your loved one's comfort remains at the forefront. Even if it's emotionally draining to imagine advanced dementia or end-of-life care, facing those realities now spares heartbreak later. A caregiver once told me, "Making these decisions before the crisis hit was the best gift I gave us all. It let us spend more time just being together, instead of drowning in paperwork when things got rough."

A Gentle Conclusion: Crafting Security and Honor

Legal documents, financial spreadsheets, and ethical quandaries can feel worlds apart from the day-to-day tasks of bathing, feeding, or reminiscing with your loved one. Yet they're deeply intertwined. Each signature, each plan, each conversation helps preserve dignity. It ensures that even in confusion, your loved one's essence isn't lost. You're not just signing forms; you're offering stability in a journey rife with unpredictability.

Margaret, the caregiver from the start, found solace once she finalized her husband George's Power of Attorney and advanced directives. She said, "It felt like a weight was lifted. Now I know I can protect him, even if he doesn't realize what's happening." That's the real power of these tools. They transform swirling anxieties into concrete plans. They turn your heartbreak into purposeful action.

As we close this chapter, know that none of this is easy. You might face resistance from family, confusion over legal jargon, or guilt about making big decisions. But by educating yourself and seeking help—whether from lawyers, financial advisors, or support groups—you can navigate it. And in so doing, you affirm that your loved one's life has value, that their well-being matters enough to handle these complex matters with courage and care.

In the chapters ahead, we'll shift focus again—venturing into the realm of self-care for caregivers, stress management, and ways to sustain your own spirit in this demanding role. Because as you guard your loved one's rights and resources, you also need to guard your own resilience. The journey continues, but now you hold a map, a compass, and a bit more confidence in guiding them safely through the forest.

SELF-CARE AND EMOTIONAL RESILIENCE

ometime last year, I visited a home where an exhausted daughter, Teresa, was folding laundry in the dimly lit living room. Her mother, diagnosed with moderate dementia, was asleep nearby. Teresa's eyes were ringed with shadows. She looked at me and whispered, "I haven't laughed in months." I could *feel* the weight in her voice. Later that afternoon, when her mother woke up confused and upset, Teresa tried to soothe her but ended up snapping at her instead. The guilt on her face was heartbreaking. It was also familiar. In my years of caring for dementia patients, I've seen that weariness etched into countless caregivers' expressions. It's a weariness that signals burnout, fraying connections, and a desperate need for rejuvenation.

Chapters past have guided us through dementia basics, daily tasks, legal frameworks, and more. Now, we turn inward. This chapter is about **you**—the caregiver who pours compassion into someone else's life, often forgetting to refill your own cup. We'll explore how to spot the earliest flickers of burnout, how to manage stress, how to build a sturdy support network, how to embrace respite care without guilt, how to juggle work and caregiving demands, and finally, how to cultivate the emotional resilience that keeps you strong through every twist in this winding journey. Let's begin, with Teresa's story still echoing in our ears, reminding us that self-care is not a luxury, but a lifeline.

WARNING SIGNS AND PREVENTION OF CAREGIVER BURNOUT

When You Realize You're Running on Fumes

Robert is probably the main person to come to mind when I think of someone driven to exhaustion by this condition. He often confessed that he'd forgotten the last time he *truly* relaxed. He had cared for his wife with late-stage dementia for years. "I can't go to sleep without worrying what'll happen if she wakes up confused," he said. Over time, he found himself snapping at neighbors, ignoring phone calls from friends. He was always tired. Food lost its taste. A gloom settled over him, making even mundane tasks feel insurmountable. That's burnout in a nutshell: a creeping state of physical, mental, and emotional fatigue that can leave you hollowed out.

Caregiver burnout often starts subtly. Maybe you're more irritable than usual, or you skip hobbies you once adored. You might sense a haze, a numbness that disconnects you from the person you're trying so hard to help. Sometimes, it surfaces as persistent headaches or stomach issues that you can't quite explain. Or perhaps your sleep is restless, haunted by to-do lists. Recognizing these signs is crucial. This is your body and mind waving tiny red flags.

Early Signals That Demand Attention

When you find yourself losing patience over trivial matters, or you realize you can't recall the last time you laughed with genuine joy, your spirit may be calling for help. Chronic irritability is a major clue. So is that sinking feeling that you're waking up to a never-ending treadmill of duties, with no finish line in sight. If you feel a persistent sense of guilt—believing you're failing your loved one or that you should always do more—you're likely flirting with burnout's edge. Physically, you might notice lingering colds or aches, as stress can weaken immunity. Emotionally, a sense of helplessness can creep in, overshadowing hope.

Intervening early is the best gift you can give yourself—and, indirectly, your loved one. Addressing burnout before it fully sets in keeps you from sliding into deeper despair. That might mean confiding in a friend, seeking professional counseling, or scheduling a checkup with your doctor. Counseling can be a haven for venting frustrations, learning coping tools, and discovering that you're not broken—just overwhelmed. Sometimes, we also underestimate the power of simple stress reduction strategies like short walks, stretching, or losing ourselves in a favorite novel. These breaks can be oxygen when you're gasping under caregiving's pressure.

Preventing the Spiral

I had another patient who came up with quite a genius idea (if perhaps incorrectly judged as selfish by many as soon as they heard it). She established "unavailable hours" each evening, even if only for 30 minutes, to drink tea on the porch or read a chapter of a mystery. It was "her" time and absolutely no one else's. She told me, "It was strange to carve out that time, but it saved my sanity." Prevention hinges on realistic boundaries—acknowledging you can't do everything. Maybe you can't attend every doctor's appointment alone or manage all the household chores. That's okay. It's also about scheduling self-care regularly. A 10-minute meditation at dawn. A Sunday call with a supportive friend. A monthly therapy session if possible.

Burnout rarely disappears on its own. Left unchecked, it can morph into chronic anxiety, depression, or a complete emotional breakdown. By spotting the patterns early and taking consistent micro-steps, you can shield yourself. And the result? A more patient, compassionate version of you emerges—the one your loved one truly needs.

STRESS MANAGEMENT TECHNIQUES

The Moment That Belongs to You

A while back, I was walking through a bustling hospital hallway. Two orderlies rushed past, pushing wheelchairs. Phones rang at the nurse's station. Yet in a corner, I noticed a caregiver—eyes closed, hands in lap— taking measured breaths. I paused in curiosity. Later, she told me she was practicing a quick mindfulness exercise, picturing a calm beach scene. "It's my secret weapon," she whispered with a smile. Sometimes, that single minute of mindful breathing is the difference between meltdown and composure.

Mindfulness is all about being present in the here and now—observing your thoughts without judging them as "good" or "bad." By centering on your breath, the rustle of your clothing, or the hum of distant chatter, you anchor yourself, letting stress slip away momentarily. Some caregivers find relief in progressive muscle relaxation: systematically tensing, then releasing, each muscle group from toes to scalp. Others prefer guided imagery. Picture yourself strolling through a peaceful forest or floating on a serene lake. The mind is powerful. A few minutes of mental stillness can reset the emotional clock.

Other Paths to Zen

There's no one-size-fits-all formula for stress management. What soothes you might irritate someone else. Some caregivers adore journaling, using pen and paper as an emotional spillway. They scribble everything: frustrations, joys, random thoughts. Others channel stress through art—finger-painting, photography, or even adult coloring books. Music can also be transformative. Play a favorite song softly in the background, or belt out a tune if that's your release. If you're more physically inclined, dancing (yes, even silly living-room dancing) can shake off tension.

The key is making these outlets part of your daily routine, not a once-in-a-blue-moon treat. Try five minutes of guided meditation every morning. Or commit to a nightly ritual of freeform journaling, no matter how tired you are. Regular practice cements these habits into your routine, building an internal reservoir of calm you can tap into when crises strike.

Gathering Resources for the Journey

We live in a digital age teeming with apps and websites. Tools like "Insight Timer," "Calm," or "Headspace" offer guided meditations you can do anywhere. Or you might find local yoga or stress reduction classes—often at community centers or senior organizations. If a formal class feels daunting, look for online courses where you can learn at your own pace. Some caregivers I know have found solace in group mindfulness sessions—virtual or in person—where they connect with others on the same path.

Keep reminding yourself: stress relief isn't indulgence, it's maintenance. Just like fueling a car or charging a phone. You can't operate on empty. If guilt nags at you for taking a break, gently remind yourself that you're recharging so you can keep giving the best possible care.

BUILDING A SUPPORT NETWORK: FINDING YOUR TRIBE

That Critical Lifeline

A caregiver once told me, "I feel like I'm stranded on an island." Maybe you've felt the same. Dementia care can be isolating, especially when friends fade away, unsure of how to help. But forging connections is essential. A solid support network can transform your daily grind into a collective effort. It might be as simple as a neighbor who brings groceries or a cousin who calls every Sunday. In those gestures, you realize you aren't as alone as you feared.

Family is often the first tier of support—siblings, adult children, or extended relatives. But families can be complicated. Sometimes, well-intentioned loved ones are too distant or busy, or they disagree on how to handle caregiving decisions. That's why broadening your circle matters. Join local or online caregiver support groups. There, you'll find people who "get it" on a visceral level. They've endured midnight confusion, hospital runs, aggressive outbursts. They offer empathy and practical advice in the same breath. Sometimes you just need someone to say, "I know exactly how that feels," to lighten your burden.

Cultivating Connections

Building a network takes initiative. Search for caregiver meetups in your city, or explore online forums if you can't leave home. Community organizations or churches often run caregiving workshops or social events. Volunteering can also connect you with like-minded folks. If you have time, consider helping at a local respite care center or participating in a charity event for dementia awareness. Oddly enough, by giving, you often receive: new friends, new coping strategies, new hope.

Never hesitate to ask for help. It might mean telling a friend, "Can you sit with Dad on Friday so I can do errands?" or emailing your child's teacher to explain you might miss some school events due to caregiving. People appreciate direct requests. They'd rather you specify how they can assist instead of hinting or staying silent. That honesty fosters deeper bonds and shows them you trust their willingness to support you.

Leaning on Your Tribe

The beauty of a strong support network is that it's dynamic. One friend might offer emotional solace via late-night texts. Another might excel at practical tasks like cooking or yard work. A coworker might share time management tips. A neighbor might provide respite by visiting your loved one once a week. With each contribution, your load lightens a bit. You also gain varied perspectives: someone might suggest a local adult day program you hadn't heard of, or a new app for medication tracking. Sharing experiences, venting frustrations, and celebrating small wins become communal acts.

A word of caution: reciprocity matters. Offer your own listening ear or help out if another caregiver needs support. That mutual exchange fosters genuine, enduring relationships. Caregiving can be all-consuming, but if you can give a bit back, you'll feel more integrated and less like a charity case. "We're in this together," one caregiver said in a group session I attended. And that's precisely how your tribe can sustain you—even on days you feel you're barely hanging on.

TAKING A BREAK WITHOUT GUILT

Easing the Pressure Valve

Respite care. The term sounds clinical, but in reality, it can be a gentle hush, a moment of stillness in the chaos. Think of it as a short vacation from your caregiving responsibilities, where someone else handles the tasks while you catch your breath. I once worked with someone who cared for her husband 24/7. She felt she was constantly on alert, never off-duty. Her sister convinced her to try a weekend respite program at a local adult day care. "I was so anxious at first," she admitted. "But after that weekend, I felt alive again. It recharged my batteries."

Respite care can take many forms. Maybe an in-home care service sends a trained professional for a few hours or overnight. Or your loved one attends an adult day care program where they interact with peers, play games, and receive supervision. Some caregivers find short-term stays at assisted living facilities. Whatever the shape, respite care offers you, the caregiver, a chance to exhale deeply, knowing your loved one is safe and tended to.

Overcoming the Guilt

Caregivers often wrestle with guilt. "How can I leave them? They need me." Or they fear their loved one might feel abandoned or become disoriented in new surroundings. It's natural to worry. But consider this: if you burn out completely, who will care for them then? Taking breaks doesn't mean you love them any less. In fact, it's an act of love—to sustain your own well-being so you can continue supporting them over the long haul.

Explain to your loved one, in simple terms, that you need a brief rest, just like they might need a nap. Reassure them you'll be back soon. If they're anxious about new people or places, you might do a gentle introduction before the respite day. A short trial run can ease everyone's nerves. And if they protest, remember that their short-term displeasure may protect both of you from bigger problems down the road.

Finding the Right Fit

Locating respite care options can take some detective work. Start by asking local senior centers, memory care facilities, or social services for recommendations. Some nonprofits or religious organizations have volunteer respite programs. Compare costs, read reviews, and if possible, visit the facility or meet the caregiver in advance. Good respite care not only benefits you but also provides enriching activities for your loved one—maybe light exercises, crafts, or gentle socialization.

Then, create a simple plan. Pack your loved one's essentials: a list of medications, emergency contacts, favorite snacks or comforting items, and any special instructions. Communicate all crucial details to the respite caregiver. The more prepared you are, the smoother the transition. And once you step away, let yourself truly rest. Use the time to sleep, watch a movie, or see a friend. Resist the urge to check in every five minutes. This is your chance to refill your emotional reservoir.

BALANCING WORK AND CAREGIVING

When You're Wearing Two Hats

Linda was a nurse by profession and a caregiver by necessity. Every morning, she raced to get her mother settled before rushing to her early shift. Lunch breaks were spent making phone calls to doctors or rearranging her mother's appointments. By evening, she felt drained, with her own tasks piling up. That push and pull can feel relentless: meeting office deadlines while also fielding calls from a home aide or frantically scheduling medication pick-ups. Work plus caregiving can equal a perfect storm—unless you find strategies to manage your day more effectively.

Practical Tactics for a Chaotic Routine

First, map out your priorities. Which tasks absolutely must happen today? Which can wait until tomorrow or be delegated? Tools like Google Calendar, Trello, or simple pen-and-paper to-do lists help you see the big picture. Some caregivers color-code tasks: red for urgent, yellow for semi-urgent, green for flexible. By visually categorizing chores, you can focus your energy on pressing matters first. And if something isn't urgent or can be handled by someone else, practice letting go.

When it comes to your job, open dialogue with your employer can be a game-changer. Discuss flexible scheduling or the possibility of partial remote work. Many workplaces have become more accommodating, recognizing that employees have personal obligations—especially in a post-pandemic world. If your organization offers employee assistance programs (EAPs), take advantage of them. They often provide counseling, legal advice, or referrals for respite care. Let your employer know that with a bit of flexibility, you can remain a productive team member while still caring for your family.

Streamlining Daily Routines

Meal prep is a godsend. Spending a couple of hours on the weekend to batch-cook meals or chop ingredients can save you from nightly chaos. Store everything in clear containers so you can quickly heat up a healthy dinner after work. Also, consider delegating tasks to other family members, or even close friends who offer help. Let your teen handle laundry. Ask a sibling to manage prescription refills. Hire a cleaning service once a month if finances allow. Small changes can carve out pockets of breathing room.

Lastly, remember to carve out mini-breaks for yourself—even in the middle of a busy day. A quick stroll around the block, five minutes of stretching, or a mental reset with a short meditation can do wonders. Don't wait until you're on the brink of meltdown to pause. Integrating these micro-breaks helps keep your stress from boiling over. In essence, balancing work and caregiving is about thoughtful planning, flexible adaptation, and relentless self-care. If Linda could find a rhythm, so can you.

STAYING STRONG IN THE FACE OF ADVERSITY

Bending Without Breaking

In the midst of caring for a dementia patient, emotional resilience is the invisible armor that shields your heart. Resilience isn't about denying pain or stress. It's about acknowledging the hardship and still believing you can handle tomorrow. I often think of one of my first ever clients Jorge, whose wife's dementia escalated quickly. Each new symptom felt like a blow. But day by day, he found small ways to cope—writing in a gratitude journal, savoring coffee in the morning sun, even praying quietly. Over months, his sorrow didn't vanish, but he discovered a deeper well of strength within.

Building That Inner Core

Emotional resilience starts with understanding that hardship is part of this journey. That acceptance frees you from feeling ambushed by every downturn. Next, find strategies that help you bounce back. Problem-solving is key: when a new issue arises—like nighttime wandering—brainstorm solutions rather than simply despairing. Maybe you install motion sensors or a bed alarm. Or rearrange the bedroom for safety. Tackle challenges systematically, focusing on what you can change.

Don't forget self-compassion. Caregiving can involve mistakes, regrets, or feeling you're never doing enough. In those moments, pause and gently remind yourself you're human. A short mantra can help: "I am doing my best, and that's good enough." Over time, this quiet encouragement seeps into your mindset, lessening harsh self-criticism.

Self-Reflection and Growth

Journaling is a powerful tool for weaving resilience. When you write down daily experiences—both frustrations and small triumphs—you gain clarity. Patterns emerge, solutions become clearer, and random thoughts transform into insight. Some caregivers also swear by meditation or quiet reflection. They find a serene corner each day to breathe and scan their emotions. This gentle check-in fosters emotional awareness, letting you catch negativity or burnout symptoms before they spiral.

Activities like gratitude exercises also reshape perspective. Consider scribbling down three things you're grateful for every evening: a neighbor's kindness, your loved one's smile at breakfast, a simple dessert you enjoyed. Over time, these micro-moments of appreciation anchor you in positivity, even when the overarching journey feels tough. Additionally, setting personal goals—like finishing a book, mastering a new recipe, or learning an instrument—injects your life with purpose beyond caregiving. Achieving incremental objectives reminds you that you're more than a caretaker. You're a whole person with dreams and capabilities.

The Bigger Picture: Fostering Sustainable Compassion

As we reach the end of this chapter, let's reflect on the mosaic of ideas we've explored. You've learned to spot the glimmers of burnout. You've discovered mindfulness techniques that can cradle your frayed nerves. You've seen how forging a support network ensures you're not bearing the weight alone. You've learned respite care can be a beacon of relief, how time management keeps you afloat, and how resilience is the bedrock of your emotional fortitude.

Caregiving is often described as a marathon, not a sprint. You need stamina, pacing, and an unwavering sense of why you embarked on this path. Yes, you're caring for someone else, but you must also care for yourself. Without self-care, the reservoir of empathy runs dry, and you risk not only your own health but the quality of life for the person you love. That's not the outcome any caregiver wants.

By integrating these strategies—small daily rituals, bigger structural supports, and a mindset of resilience—you safeguard both your well-being and theirs. You remind yourself that each day, each moment, can hold sparks of joy, no matter how deeply dementia's shadows fall. Teresa, from earlier in this chapter, found that once she prioritized short "me-moments"—painting watercolors, sharing burdens with a friend—she rediscovered laughter. Her mother's condition didn't magically improve, but Teresa's spirit did. And that shift made all the difference.

Now, as we prepare to journey into the next phase—where we'll explore advanced topics in caregiving, community resources, or perhaps new expansions on daily challenges—hold tight to the lessons here. Remember that self-care is never selfish. It's an essential scaffold, propping up your ability to give, to nurture, to love. Without it, the entire structure can collapse. So go ahead: take that break, reach out for help, breathe in the quiet hush of a mindful moment. You deserve it, and your loved one deserves a caregiver who is whole, hopeful, and fully alive.

LEVERAGING SUPPORT SYSTEMS AND RESOURCES

I t was late afternoon when I dropped by to see Darius, a caregiver who'd been tending to his father for nearly a year. He stood in the kitchen, washing dishes with trembling hands. When I asked how he was doing, he forced a smile. "Just fine," he said, but his eyes told a different story. He was isolated. Exhausted. Longing for a break from the relentless routine. That conversation stuck with me. So many caregivers, just like Darius, carry the weight alone because they don't realize there's help waiting —often just around the corner, or maybe a few clicks away.

This chapter is about building those bridges of help: finding the groups, programs, people, and resources that lift you out of isolation. We've touched on self-care, daily tasks, and the emotional resilience needed to stay afloat in the face of dementia's challenges. Now it's time to widen the lens. Because no caregiver should feel they must handle everything themselves. The world, it turns out, is brimming with allies—from local community centers to digital forums, from volunteer networks to professional services. Let's dive into these support systems that exist for you and your loved one.

FINDING AND JOINING SUPPORT GROUPS

More Than a Meeting—A Lifeline

A friend of mine was skeptical about attending her first caregiver support group. She told me, "I'm not one for talking about my problems in front of strangers." But after her mother's dementia advanced, she felt cornered by endless questions and frustrations. Finally, she took the plunge. The following week, she emerged from the community center brimming with relief. "They get it," she whispered. "I don't have to explain every detail—they already know." That's the magic of a good support group: it's not just a meeting. It's a safe haven where shared experiences form an instant bond.

Support groups offer emotional healing and practical know-how. You can learn about new medication regimens, easy mealtime hacks, or tricks for handling repetitive questions. You also hear stories of perseverance that spark hope. People share tearful confessions, triumphant breakthroughs, or simply that day's meltdown moment. The group listens, nods, and responds with empathy. It's a place to be real, to set aside the mask of "everything's fine" and say, "I'm overwhelmed." And in that honesty, healing begins.

Locating the Right Group

How do you find these circles of comfort? Start local. Community centers or hospitals often host caregiver groups. Check bulletin boards, ask staff, or browse community newsletters. Some senior agencies maintain lists of ongoing meetups. If in-person gatherings feel tricky (maybe due to your loved one's care schedule), consider online platforms. Facebook, for instance, has numerous private caregiver groups, each with its own vibe and membership rules. Meetup.com might also list local gatherings—some meet physically, others virtually. Both have their perks: face-to-face connections can feel more intimate, while online discussions let you join from home in pajamas.

Once you spot a few options, do a little research. What's the group size? Some folks thrive in large groups with diverse perspectives. Others prefer smaller, tighter-knit circles. Is there a facilitator? A structured format can keep sessions on track, while informal groups allow free-flowing conversation. Also, think about the group's focus: do they center on dementia in general, or specifically on Alzheimer's, Lewy body, or another type? Do they lean heavily on religious or spiritual perspectives, or remain secular?

Matching a group's style with your personal preferences fosters a more meaningful connection.

Making the Most of Your Group Experience

Okay, you've found "the one." You attend your first meeting—heart pounding, probably worried about being judged or having to spill your innermost frustrations. Breathe. Remember, everyone there has walked a similar path. They understand the heartbreak and hilarity that can coexist in dementia care. So speak up. Share that story about your father who wanders at night or your aunt who confuses her mirror with a window. The more you open up, the deeper the group can support you.

Also consider how you can give back. Maybe you have a tip about rummaging boxes (for fidgeting hands) or a clever bath-time trick. Offering your own wisdom not only helps others but also reminds you that your experiences hold value. If the group organizes events—like a potluck, a fundraiser, or a special speaker session—try to get involved. This fosters friendships beyond those meeting rooms. Over time, you may find yourself forging bonds that last well outside the group setting.

COMMUNITY PROGRAMS AND SERVICES: WHAT'S AVAILABLE?

Finding Community Right Where You Live

Gina is a current client of mine; she's a mother of three, juggling a full-time job and the care of her grandmother, who has advanced dementia. Gina's told me she feels like she is always two steps behind: missing kids' soccer games, skipping her own doctor appointments. In the last few weeks, she has discovered that her local senior center runs a day program for people with cognitive impairments. They have crafts, gentle exercise sessions, music therapy, etc. Best of all, Gina can now drop off her grandmother in a safe environment, go to work, and pick her up later in the day, relaxed and smiling. It has been an absolute game-changer.

Senior centers often host a variety of activities. Some have "memory cafés" where caregivers and patients can gather for coffee, conversation, and structured social time. Others coordinate bus trips or group outings. Meanwhile, nonprofits might run educational workshops on topics like legal planning, stress relief, or advanced directives. Keep an eye out for free or low-cost respite programs, too. Many nonprofits partner with local agencies to offer short-term care, giving you a window to rest.

Taking the First Step

Start by calling local agencies on aging—they typically have rosters of community offerings. Hospitals and clinics might also maintain directories. In some towns, libraries double as community hubs, listing upcoming events or hosting caregiver fairs. Try searching online with phrases like "dementia support services [your town]" or "adult day programs near me." Once you find something interesting, reach out. Ask about enrollment procedures, schedules, and fees. Some programs require an evaluation or a waiting list. Register in advance if needed, so you're not scrambling last minute.

Why It's Worth It

Community programs can break isolation, both for you and your loved one. They might join an art therapy class while you attend a parallel caregiver workshop. You'll connect with neighbors facing similar challenges. You'll learn new coping strategies from experts and from each other. Socializing is also a boon for patients—stimulation, gentle activities, maybe even new friendships. That can ease restlessness or depression. Meanwhile, you get a breather, or at least a shared sense of support. It's not an overstatement to say such programs can restore a sense of normalcy in lives tilted by dementia.

Real-Life Success Stories

I recall one caregiver retreat: a weekend getaway in a scenic lodge where caregivers met for group discussions, yoga sessions, and scenic walks. One man confided that it was the first time he'd relaxed in years. Another participant discovered a passion for watercolor painting while her spouse engaged in music therapy. That weekend, they both returned home recharged and with fresh perspectives. Another time, a local dementia-friendly fair showcased technology tools (like GPS trackers and specialized apps like My House of Memories and Mindmate) and introduced families to volunteer networks. Caregivers left brimming with ideas to simplify daily routines. These success stories highlight the powerful ripple effect of community engagement—when communities step up, caregivers can breathe easier.

DIGITAL SUPPORT NETWORKS

A World of Advice, At Your Fingertips

Not everyone can commute to a support group or day program. Some of you might be homebound, living rurally, or simply juggling too many responsibilities. That's where online resources shine. Imagine you're up at 2 AM because your loved one's experiencing sundowning confusion. You open your laptop or phone and jump into a dementia caregiver forum. Within minutes, someone across the country shares an idea: a soothing playlist, a calm voice, a light snack. Another user says, "I'm awake too—let's talk." It's a lifeline in the darkest hours.

Platforms like the Alzheimer's Association online community or Aging-Care forums connect you with caregivers globally. You'll encounter threads on everything: medication side effects, how to handle wandering, how to keep communication positive despite memory loss. You can also find specialized groups on Facebook, some private, some public, each with its own vibe. If you prefer anonymity, look for forums that let you post under a username. The key is finding a warm, moderated environment. Trolls or misinformation can lurk online, so choose reputable boards or websites affiliated with recognized organizations.

Navigating the Pitfalls

Online communities can be a godsend, but caution is warranted. Not everyone offering advice is an expert—some might share unverified remedies or vent personal frustrations. Always cross-check critical information with reliable medical sources or consult a healthcare professional. Also, be mindful of privacy. It's tempting to vent about your loved one's condition, but revealing personal data can compromise security. Use pseudonyms or limit identifying details. If a platform lacks moderation or respectful discourse, consider leaving. Support networks thrive on empathy and understanding, not drama.

Making the Most of Digital Communities

To truly benefit, engage actively. Lurking (just reading) can be helpful, but posting questions or experiences fosters deeper connections. "Hey, has anyone tried calming aromatherapy at night?" might lead to a flurry of responses. Contribute your own success stories—maybe you discovered a brilliant trick for redirecting aggression or a brand-new puzzle game that rekindles interest. This reciprocity nourishes the forum's collective wisdom.

You might also join multiple groups, each addressing a different aspect. One might focus on general dementia care. Another might revolve around a specific stage or type of dementia. A third could concentrate on caregiver mental health. Over time, you'll refine your online routine. Maybe you check in daily with a small group of digital friends who truly get your struggles. Or perhaps you only log on when a crisis arises. However you approach it, these digital networks can serve as round-the-clock shoulders to lean on, bridging distances and time zones.

PROFESSIONAL HELP: WHEN AND HOW TO SEEK IT

Calling in the Experts

I remember a caregiver named Beatriz who reached a breaking point. Her mother's dementia had escalated to frequent nighttime wandering and bouts of paranoia. Beatriz tried everything—locking doors, rearranging furniture, soothing evening routines. Nothing worked. Finally, she consulted a geriatric care manager who evaluated the home environment and her mother's needs, then devised a comprehensive plan. That included coordinating with a social worker to explore financial assistance for in-home support. Within weeks, the situation had stabilized.

Sometimes, your best efforts aren't enough. That's okay—no one can shoulder it all. Professionals like geriatric care managers bring specialized knowledge about dementia-related resources, living arrangements, and medical coordination. Social workers can guide you through insurance complexities, government benefits, and emotional hurdles. Counselors or therapists can help you process grief and stress. And if your loved one's behavior or medical status hits a perplexing snag, a neurologist or geriatric psychiatrist might be the next step.

Recognizing the Tipping Point

How do you know it's time for professional intervention? Maybe you feel perpetually overwhelmed, borderline paralyzed by daily tasks. Or your loved one's symptoms become unmanageable—violent outbursts, dramatic cognitive decline, severe depression. If you can't keep up with medical appointments or you find yourself ignoring your own health, that's a red flag. Another clue: if friends or relatives express concern for your well-being, listen closely. Sometimes, an outside perspective alerts you to hidden danger signs.

Choosing the Right Specialist

Selecting the best expert can be daunting. Start by asking your primary care doctor for a referral. They often have networks of recommended specialists. Consider the professional's credentials, yes, but also trust your gut about whether their personality aligns with your loved one's needs. A geriatric care manager might coordinate everything from medication reviews to home safety checks. A mental health counselor might focus on emotional resilience. Don't hesitate to meet with several candidates. You deserve a comfortable, trusting partnership.

The Impact of Expert Intervention

Professional help can lift an immense burden. You'll gain practical advice tailored to your unique situation. Maybe they'll suggest a new medication or behavioral therapy approach. Perhaps they'll connect you with a day program or help you find a specialized memory care unit if needed. Just the knowledge that someone else is in your corner can ease that lonely feeling of "it's all on me." Meanwhile, your loved one benefits from more cohesive care. Experts bring a neutral perspective, spotting issues you might miss due to emotional involvement. Together, you'll craft a plan that fosters safety, dignity, and a better quality of life for everyone involved.

EXPANDING YOUR SUPPORT TEAM

The Power of a Helping Hand

I meet many male caregivers who are usually hunched over the stove, cooking dinner, while their wives, who have dementia, wander restlessly in the living room. On one occasion, I was on an impromptu home visit, and it was quite the assault on the senses. The phone was ringing, the dog was barking, and chaos swirled around the household. Suddenly, a knock at the door: a volunteer from a local organization who'd come to keep his wife company for a couple of hours. The man exhaled, eyes tearing up. "I didn't realize how badly I needed this break," he said. That's the beauty of volunteers. They can inject a ray of calm into your storm.

Volunteers do more than just lighten your load. They offer companionship for your loved one—someone to chat with, take a walk alongside, or solve simple puzzles with. That social interaction can ease agitation and brighten mood. Volunteers might also handle light chores, run errands, or help with mealtime tasks. Meanwhile, you can step away to rest, run to the store, or simply breathe.

Finding and Recruiting Volunteers

Look first to local volunteer organizations, such as nonprofits focused on senior care or your place of worship if you're active in a faith community. They often have rosters of vetted volunteers eager to help. Sometimes, high school or college students volunteer for community service hours, bringing fresh energy and a willingness to learn. Another approach is to post a notice on community boards or online forums: "Seeking volunteer companion for an elder with dementia." Just be sure to screen respondents. Ask for references or do a quick interview. You want someone reliable and caring.

Once you welcome a volunteer, define roles clearly. Do you want them to read aloud, play a board game, or help with housekeeping? Let them know your loved one's quirks: maybe they love big-band music but hate loud TV. That clarity sets everyone up for success.

Hiring In-Home Aides

Beyond volunteers, consider professional in-home aides. They bring training, experience, and a deeper skill set—especially if your loved one needs help with bathing, dressing, or medical tasks. In-home aides can often accommodate flexible schedules, from a few hours a week to full-time. This support can be invaluable if you need to work or simply catch up on errands. The cost varies, but some insurance policies or Medicaid programs might cover part of it.

As with volunteers, communication is key. Outline expected duties, from medication reminders to meal prep. Share any special instructions about mobility or cognitive issues. Maintaining open communication fosters trust and ensures the aide understands your loved one's preferences. If possible, schedule a trial shift to observe how the aide and your loved one interact. If there's rapport and respect, you're on the right track.

Creating a Caregiving Team

Volunteers and aides aren't just extra hands; they're part of a larger support network. You might also have family members rotating visits or neighbors who check in. Make sure everyone stays in the loop. Maybe keep a shared notebook or digital app where you jot down daily notes—moods, meal logs, medication changes. Encourage feedback. If a volunteer notices your loved one gets restless around dusk, that's valuable info to share with the aide. A cohesive team thrives on collaboration, not duplication or confusion. By weaving volunteers and professionals into your life, you free yourself from being the sole pillar. And that, in turn, helps both you and your loved one flourish.

NAVIGATING HEALTHCARE SYSTEMS

Becoming Their Voice

When Paula's father was rushed to the hospital for a fall, she found herself surrounded by medical staff who rattled off terms like "CT scan," "contusion," "neuro consult," all while her father stared blankly. She felt lost in the jargon. But she took a deep breath, grabbed a notebook, and asked the doctor to slow down. She repeated questions for clarity, scribbled down each answer, and made sure to mention her father's dementia so they'd adapt their communication. In that moment, Paula realized: she was his advocate. She had to ensure he got the best possible care, and that his dignity remained intact.

As a caregiver, you stand on the front lines of healthcare, bridging the gap between your loved one's needs and a complex medical system. You coordinate appointments, gather medication lists, and interpret signs and symptoms. You note changes in mood, appetite, or physical ability. That knowledge is gold. It can guide physicians toward better diagnoses or prompt them to reconsider treatments. Your role is vital. Don't underestimate the power of your observations.

Key Advocacy Skills

Preparing for doctor visits is half the battle. Create a concise list of questions: "He seems more disoriented after dinner—could it be medication timing?" or "She's refusing to eat certain foods—should we consider a swallowing evaluation?" Keep a journal of daily patterns—sleep, agitation, appetite—to share at appointments. This data paints a clearer picture for healthcare providers. If the medical language feels overwhelming, ask them to rephrase. They're there to help, not to confuse.

Managing time and resources can be tricky—often there are multiple specialists, from neurologists to physical therapists. If scheduling becomes dizzying, see if a geriatric care manager or social worker can coordinate. Or harness digital tools like a shared online calendar. Additionally, learning basic medical terms or reading about your loved one's condition can empower you to ask sharper questions. The more you grasp, the less likely you are to feel steamrolled during appointments.

Overcoming Common Obstacles

Healthcare systems can be labyrinthine, with insurance forms, waiting lists, and conflicting advice. You might face endless phone tag just to schedule an MRI. Or a doctor who seems hurried, skipping over your concerns. Advocate firmly yet politely. If you sense your loved one isn't receiving appropriate attention, request a second opinion. If hospital staff aren't adopting dementia-friendly practices, speak up. Sometimes, contacting a patient advocate within the hospital or clinic can expedite solutions.

If you need extra guidance, consider patient advocacy workshops. They teach negotiation, effective communication, and medical literacy. Many nonprofits or caregiver coalitions host such events. Online resources can also walk you through insurance intricacies or explain medical procedures in plain language. The more you equip yourself, the more effectively you can champion your loved one's well-being.

Bringing Compassion to Every Interaction

Remember, advocacy isn't about clashing with healthcare professionals. It's about collaboration. Approach doctors, nurses, or therapists with respect. They hold clinical expertise; you hold daily-lived expertise of your loved one. Together, you form a powerful team. If something feels off, voice it. If a nurse does something particularly kind, acknowledge it. Positive relationships in healthcare can smooth future interactions and encourage staff to go the extra mile.

As your loved one's advocate, you channel compassion into action. You safeguard them from potential oversights, ensuring quality and continuity of care. It can be emotionally taxing—witnessing medical decline or absorbing disheartening news. But it also offers a sense of purpose. You're their voice when they can't speak, their defender in an often impersonal system. In that role, you embody the beating heart of caregiving: unwavering love backed by steadfast resolve.

· · ·

A Gentle Close: Tapping Into a Network of Hope

As we wrap up this chapter on leveraging support systems and resources, let's return to Darius, the caregiver from the beginning. Soon after our conversation, he found a local support group, hired a volunteer for occasional companionship, and explored adult day care options at a nearby senior center. He told me, months later, that his entire outlook shifted. "I'm not alone. My dad and I are part of a bigger circle," he said. And that circle—composed of fellow caregivers, community initiatives, digital allies, professionals, and volunteers—continues to sustain him.

You, too, can build such a circle. Reach out, even if it feels awkward at first. Try a group meeting, explore an online forum, call a volunteer organization. Investigate respite programs or professional services. Rally siblings, neighbors, and friends. It's not about burdening others; it's about weaving a supportive net where no single strand bears the entire load. Because dementia caregiving isn't meant to be tackled in solitude. The resources are out there, waiting for you to take that first, brave step.

In the chapters to come, we'll venture further into advanced strategies, future planning, and perhaps more nuanced emotional territories. But for now, hold onto this idea: help is everywhere. You simply have to invite it in. And once you do, you'll breathe a little easier, walk a little steadier, and realize that yes—there is a whole community behind you, cheering you on every step of the way.

INSPIRATIONAL STORIES AND LESSONS LEARNED

I n the last 25 years, I've met countless people going through the same
journey that you are going through. And it's because of all these countless interactions that I can confidently say that you never really know
how strong you are until you're tested. That's what I once told a caregiver
named Yvonne, who looked ready to crumble under the weight of her
father's new diagnosis. She'd spent weeks guiding him through a haze of
confusion, alternating between fear and frustration. Over tea one afternoon, I
said, "Sometimes, the worst moments reveal the best in us." Her eyes
watered at the notion. Yet, a few months later, she proved it true, stepping up
in ways she never thought she could. This chapter is about moments like
that. It's about caregivers who've navigated crisis after crisis and discovered
that resilience is more than survival—it's transformation. We'll share their
stories, glean their lessons, and uncover how joy, growth, and a shift in
perspective can light even the darkest paths.

OVERCOMING CAREGIVING CHALLENGES

The Phone Call No One Expects

I had a client who told me that she was midway through an early
morning shift at the bakery when her phone buzzed. A neighbor's frantic

voice told her that her mother, who had moderate-stage dementia, had wandered out in her pajamas and gotten lost. In that dizzying moment, my client realized life would never be the same. She was a single parent with limited income, living in a cramped studio apartment. "I didn't have extra money for fancy care facilities," she confided, tears brimming. "But I know I get sh*t done so it's going to happen one way or another."

From day one, it felt like she was juggling glass marbles on a tightrope. Her mother's needs grew daily, from bathroom assistance to constant reminders about everything from mealtimes to basic hygiene. But she refused to let circumstances crush her. She discovered a few local nonprofits that offered small grants for medical supplies—things like adult incontinence products or a walker. She tapped a church charity for partial rent support. And she learned to repurpose everyday items to keep her mother engaged: turning an old photo album into a memory game, or using color-coded bins to reduce confusion about where essentials belonged.

Her biggest triumph, though, was building a circle of allies. One neighbor, who'd initially been a stranger, offered to check on her mother during the day whilst she was at work. Another friend took on the role of "meal buddy," dropping off simple dinners when she worked late. "I realized I wasn't alone," she told me. "I just had to let people in." Through creative problem-solving, dogged resource-hunting, and that unwavering grit, she transformed daily chaos into a stable routine. Yes, it was still tough. But she found her resilience humming beneath the weariness.

Family in Flux: The Sudden Shift

The Thompson clan—Adam, Sophia, and their teenage twins—had prided themselves on being a team for everything. Family dinners, weekend movie nights, volunteering together. Then, seemingly overnight, their grandmother's dementia took a sharp turn. One day she was managing her own meals; the next, she was wandering the house at odd hours, unable to recall which room was hers. Everyone scrambled. Sophia rearranged her home office to create a makeshift bedroom on the ground floor. Adam handled finances, investigating Medicaid coverage and local adult day programs. The twins pitched in with chores, cooking, or simply sitting and chatting with Grandma when she felt anxious.

"At first, it felt like our world flipped upside down," Adam admitted. "But we soon found we were stronger together." They learned to adapt by communicating openly: nightly check-ins at the dinner table, sharing concerns or bright spots. They tapped neighbors for respite or advice. They discovered the local synagogue offered caregiver support sessions and embraced that sense of community. Over time, they realized each new challenge forced them to flex their problem-solving muscles. When grandmother refused to bathe, they tried music therapy in the bathroom—singing old tunes from her youth—to gently coax her into the shower. It worked. The Thompson family's story underlines how resilience often blooms in the soil of collaboration. They didn't handle everything perfectly, but they faced each blow with a unified front. And that solidarity fueled them.

The Emotional Journey of Resilience

Both Brenda's and the Thompsons' stories highlight the roller-coaster of emotions that come with caregiving. Doubt creeps in at odd hours, making you question your abilities. Perseverance answers back, reminding you of reasons to keep going. Guilt, frustration, even flashes of anger swirl in your mind. But woven among those low moments are flickers of triumph: a day without a meltdown, a small glimmer of recognition in your loved one's eyes, or a new strategy that finally works.

Over and over, caregivers describe resilience as something that formed when they had no other choice. They discovered an inner reservoir of grit. They found pockets of grace. And in forging that path, they impacted not just their own well-being, but also the life quality of their loved one. A calmer, more prepared caregiver often leads to calmer, more grounded patient experiences. It's an upward spiral. That's the magic of resilience: once it takes root, it keeps growing, shaping better futures for everyone involved.

WISDOM AND ADVICE FROM EXPERIENCED CAREGIVERS

Harvesting Decades of Insight

Imagine a lively roundtable in a community hall, with a half-dozen caregivers who've each been in the trenches for years. Some cared for parents, others for spouses. All have war stories to tell. They speak of heartbreak, learning curves, and triumphs that taste sweeter than any normal victory could. Over time, these caregivers compiled a mental ledger of do's and don'ts that can save newcomers from reinventing the wheel.

One of the biggest lessons? Patience is gold. Expect that your loved one may ask the same question twenty times an hour. Accept that you can't re-explain reality into them if their mind is stuck. Instead, meet them where they are—gently, kindly, without letting frustration overshadow love. Another lesson is flexibility. Dementia rarely follows a neat schedule. Good days and bad days can swap without warning. "You learn to adapt, to keep Plan B and Plan C ready," said a good friend of mine, who'd pivoted to a new routine whenever her mother's behavior shifted. These are the twin pillars of effective care: patience and flexibility.

Practical Strategies for Immediate Use

Those same seasoned caregivers champion the value of establishing a daily routine. Structure lowers anxiety for many dementia patients. Maybe at 9 AM it's breakfast, at 11 AM a short walk, at 2 PM an art activity, and so forth. The predictability can reduce confusion and outbursts. But don't become overly rigid—some days, you'll need to shuffle tasks around.

They also stress self-care. One longtime caregiver, Harold, confessed he neglected his own health for months, skipping doctor visits because he couldn't bear leaving his wife. He eventually developed serious fatigue and borderline depression. Through counseling, he realized caring for himself wasn't selfish; it was essential to stay functional. He now schedules short breaks each day to read, sip tea, or walk around the block. "I come back more patient and less reactive," he observed. The irony is that by stepping away, you often return a better caregiver.

How Caregiving Has Evolved

In decades past, caregivers might have acted reactively: waiting for crises, then scrambling. Now, many approach it proactively, anticipating needs before they become emergencies. That can mean setting up legal documents early, scouting adult day programs in advance, or preparing a respite care rotation plan. Technology has also altered the caregiving landscape. Some caregivers use medication reminder apps or wearable trackers that alert them if their loved one wanders too far. Others rely on video calls to keep distant relatives in the loop. The key is to remain open to new ideas. As one caregiver joked, "I used to be a technophobe. Now I'm scanning grocery lists and scheduling everything online. It's worth it!"

Nuggets of Wisdom and Encouragement

Caregivers pass around inspirational quips like tokens of solidarity. One popular mantra is "The small victories are the big victories." Did your loved one spontaneously recall your name today? That's a reason to celebrate. I had another caregiver recall the moment her father recognized an old family photo and smiled, calling her by a childhood nickname. It was fleeting. But that fleeting connection fueled her for weeks. These stories remind us that in the fog of dementia, every beam of clarity or comfort matters deeply.

Anecdotes of unexpected joy pop up too. A caregiver's mother, who rarely spoke, suddenly joined in a silly dance upon hearing a favorite old tune. A father, thought too frail to enjoy anything, burst into laughter at a grandchild's puppet show. Such glimpses break the monotony of routine care and rekindle hope. They also illustrate the bond between caregiver and patient can still blossom, even in the midst of decline.

FINDING JOY IN THE SMALL VICTORIES

Choosing to See the Bright Spots

One caregiver, Marisol, told me she used to dwell on everything going wrong. Her mother's repeated questions grated on her nerves. The mounting chores suffocated her free time. Then she stumbled on a simple trick: every evening, she wrote down one positive moment from the day. Sometimes it was a tiny breakthrough—Mom tying her shoelaces unaided, or finishing a puzzle. Gradually, these nightly reflections shifted Marisol's mindset. "I realized how many sweet moments we actually had."

It can be easy to get buried under the strain. But focusing on small achievements changes the narrative. Maybe you managed to calm an outburst with a new tactic. Or your loved one finally slept through the night. Or you found a more comfortable wheelchair cushion. Each success is a building block of optimism. Collectively, they bolster resilience, reminding you that progress, even if slow, is real.

Stories of Joy and Success

Tanya's father had all but lost the ability to speak. She grew desperate for a way to connect. One day, a visiting friend strummed a guitar, playing an old folk song. Her father's eyes lit up, and he began tapping his foot in rhythm. Tanya almost burst into tears. That simple moment—seeing him respond—flooded her with joy. She now hosts "mini concerts" once a week, inviting neighbors who play instruments. Even if her father can't talk, the music sparks a glint in his eyes. It's these glimpses of joy that reaffirm caregiving can be more than chores and stress—it can be a shared journey of discovery.

Reconnecting with family can also yield surprising happiness. A caregiver named Dave decided to host small, low-key get-togethers where extended family pitched in. One cousin always baked brownies, an aunt brought old photos to reminisce over. They formed a supportive circle, and Dave's mother often beamed at the chatter. In these gatherings, he saw that while the disease chipped away at some aspects of life, it also illuminated the power of unity and love. And that realization was euphoric.

Gratitude as a Caregiving Superpower

A daily gratitude practice can shift your entire emotional climate. Maybe you note three things you're grateful for: a hot cup of coffee, a neighbor who dropped off soup, a quiet half hour to read. Over time, this practice rewires your perspective. Even on days overshadowed by new medical complications, you'll find tiny blessings. This undercurrent of thankfulness fosters a more positive environment for you and your loved one. They feel your calm presence, sense your hopeful attitude, and respond accordingly.

Encouraging everyone in the household to adopt micro-gratitude moments can further amplify the effect. Could you share "one thing I'm thankful for today" at dinner? Or tape sticky notes of gratitude on the fridge? Remember, joy can be cultivated. It might not come naturally in the midst of exhaustion, but with gentle persistence, those small seeds can bloom into a more uplifting daily life.

Building a Joyful Inventory

Some caregivers keep a "Joy List" posted on the wall. This list might include playing an old record, flipping through a family photo album, or calling an old friend for a quick chat. Others find humor keeps them afloat—watching a short comedy clip or telling silly jokes. Laughter has a magical power to diffuse tension. Intentional acts of levity, even if brief, can remind you that life hasn't lost its sweetness entirely. When you're knee-deep in heavy tasks, these mini-retreats of joy keep you going, fueling your compassion and stamina.

PERSONAL GROWTH THROUGH CAREGIVING

A Journey of Skills and Competencies

People often assume caregiving is purely about sacrifice. Yet so many discover new talents in the process. Consider Jed, who once disliked cooking but had to learn fast when his wife's condition prevented her from preparing meals. Over time, he became a whiz at making nutritious, easy-to-eat dishes. He found himself experimenting with pureed soups, frittatas, and oatmeal bakes. To his surprise, Jed enjoyed the creativity of it. That new skill also boosted his confidence. He joked, "If this dementia journey ends, at least I'll emerge as a half-decent chef."

Others speak of improved communication and de-escalation techniques. When a loved one's behavior becomes unpredictable, caregivers learn to sense emotional shifts early. They practice calm tones, gentle touches, or a quick mental pivot to distract from frustration. These methods pay off in other areas of life—arguments with siblings, negotiations at work, or even handling moody teenagers. Being a caregiver inadvertently shapes you into a more resourceful, empathetic human being.

Unexpected Benefits and Strengthened Bonds

Caregiving also nurtures emotional depths. Many caregivers reflect that before this role, they never realized how deeply they could feel for another person. Navigating heartbreak, confusion, and fleeting triumphs fosters a kind of radical empathy. They see the world through the lens of vulnerability, recognizing how precarious and precious life is. For some, relationships with siblings or extended family strengthen as everyone bands together. Sure, conflicts can arise, but the overarching cause draws them closer. They share the load, exchange updates, unify around a parent's comfort.

In some cases, caring for someone with dementia mends old wounds. Perhaps a father and son who rarely spoke find themselves forced into daily collaboration. Over months, they break through longstanding resentment and discover they can function as a supportive team. Another caregiver told me that she and her older sister, estranged for years, reconnected over a shared desire to ease their mother's final chapter. Their mother's illness, iron-ically, became a bridge for healing.

Self-Discovery and Reflection

It's common for caregivers to experience profound introspection. Early on, one might focus only on tasks—medications, appointments, bills. But as time passes, quiet moments occur. You watch your loved one sleep, or you drive home after a tough day. In those lulls, your mind wanders, questioning your priorities. You may realize life's pace is too frantic. Or maybe you see how resilience has always been part of you, just waiting to surface. Some caregivers realize they've developed a calmer, kinder approach to conflict, which trickles into all relationships.

Journaling can crystallize these reflections. Even scribbling down a few lines about how the day went—what triggered tears, what sparked a laugh—can highlight personal growth. Over weeks, patterns emerge. Maybe you spot recurring triggers and become adept at sidestepping them. Or you discover your best coping times are the quiet early mornings. This self-awareness leads to a deeper sense of identity. Caregiving, in that sense, becomes more than an obligation; it's a catalyst for personal evolution.

Testimonials of Transformation

Zoe, who cared for her uncle, discovered she was unusually adept at medical research. She later pivoted into a new job as a patient advocate. "It's not just a job," she told me. "It's a calling born from everything I learned helping Uncle Rick." Another caregiver overcame her lifelong fear of public speaking because she started running monthly support group sessions for her community. She found her voice, literally, in the process. These stories underscore that the darkest valleys can lead to surprising peaks. Caregiving can be a crucible that forges unexpected strengths, forging new roads for your future.

STAYING POSITIVE THROUGH STRUGGLES

Reframing the Challenge

Not long ago, I met a caregiver named Mika who faced relentless setbacks: recurring hospital stays, mounting bills, unpredictable mood swings from her grandmother. Yet Mika seemed buoyed by an undercurrent of optimism. "Don't get me wrong," she said. "I have meltdowns, but I always try to see a doorway instead of a dead end." She focused on small increments of progress—like her grandmother's mild improvement in appetite after a medication tweak. Each glimmer convinced Mika there was a path forward. That mental pivot helped her avoid drowning in negativity.

She was living proof that perspective is a powerful tool: seeing setbacks as catalysts for problem-solving, rather than walls.

Techniques for a Positive Mindset

Practicing positive self-talk is one approach. Instead of scolding yourself for mistakes, remind yourself you're learning as you go. If your loved one refuses to cooperate, you might say, "I did my best today. Tomorrow we'll try something new." Affirmations might feel cheesy at first—whispering "I'm capable" in the mirror—but they can anchor your attitude when storms rage. Setting realistic goals also helps you celebrate incremental wins. Maybe your goal for the week is to finalize one medical appointment and try a new stress-relief method. Achieving these micro-goals fuels confidence, which in turn cultivates positivity.

Real Stories of Positive Transformation

Terry's mother rarely recognized him by name. At first, that crushed him. He'd slump into despair each time she asked, "Who are you?" But he realized dwelling on that heartbreak wasn't helping. So he shifted his focus. He celebrated that she still smiled at him, enjoying his presence. He introduced himself in a playful manner—"Hey, I'm your favorite dance partner!"—turning repeated confusion into a bit of fun. Over time, that consistent positivity soothed his mother, who then responded better to daily tasks. It didn't fix everything, but it made the journey less sorrowful.

Caregivers who adopt a hopeful stance often notice improved cooperation from their loved ones. A calm, upbeat voice can reduce tension. Conversely, negative energy sometimes fuels agitation or anxiety in someone with dementia. That's not to blame caregivers for being upset (your feelings are valid), but it illustrates how your emotional climate can influence theirs. Indeed, positivity and hope aren't just for your own sanity—they can ripple outward, shaping the caregiving dynamic.

How It Boosts Caregiving Outcomes

When you consistently approach challenges with a "we'll figure this out" mindset, you're more likely to brainstorm creative solutions and persist through trial and error. This openness fosters a stable environment. Your loved one senses they're cared for by someone who believes in improvement or at least in comfort. Over time, you may see fewer behavioral flare-ups, as your empathy and calm presence reduce stress triggers. Also, you'll find your own satisfaction rising, even if external circumstances remain tough. A sense of purpose emerges from each day's small but meaningful triumphs, fueling your dedication.

MOVING FORWARD: EMBRACING THE ROLE OF A CAREGIVER

Accepting the Caregiving Journey

It's easy to resent the relentless demands of caregiving, to long for your old life. But acceptance can shift the emotional landscape. Simone, a nurse by profession, once told me she fought the idea of becoming her father's care-giver for months, feeling it overshadowed her identity. Then, after reading a memoir by another caregiver, something clicked. She said, "I stopped seeing it as an interruption and began viewing it as a chapter in our story." Embracing the caregiver role doesn't erase the challenges—it simply reframes them as a responsibility that can hold meaning, lessons, and even unexpected joys.

Stories of Empowerment

I recall a caregiver named Marcus who, initially shy about confrontation, found himself advocating fiercely for his wife's right to specialized therapy. He negotiated with insurance reps, wrote letters to the local health board, and even spoke at a public hearing about dementia care. "I never thought I'd have that kind of courage," he marveled. "But doing it for her made me unstoppable." In stepping into that advocacy role, Marcus not only helped his wife but grew into a more confident, purposeful version of himself. That's the flip side of caregiving's burdens: it can spark leadership qualities, empathy, and a sense of personal agency you never knew you possessed.

The Long-Term Impact on Identity

Caregiving, especially for dementia, can last years. Over that span, it alters your sense of self. Some incorporate it fully, describing themselves as "a caregiver who also works in marketing" or "a parent who also looks after my mother." Others hold it more quietly, but still feel the transformation. The key is not letting caregiving eclipse every other aspect of who you are. You're still someone with hobbies, dreams, social connections. The goal is integra-tion rather than overshadowing. The caregiver identity becomes one thread among many in your life.

That said, many reflect that caregiving introduced them to a deeper well of compassion or reshaped their career path. Maybe you discover a knack for counseling others in similar situations and eventually volunteer for a helpline or pivot into a social work program. Or you might realize your capacity to handle stress is far greater than you imagined, which could guide you to new challenges in life. The point is, caregiving can be a crucible for growth, forging strengths that remain with you long after your duties end.

Continuing with Confidence

So how do you keep going with self-assurance rather than dread? Set future goals—maybe it's ensuring your loved one can safely remain at home for another six months, or completing advanced care directives if not already in place. Picture where you want to be personally, too. Is it possible to plan a short getaway or a sabbatical at some point? Could you build a career around the skills you've acquired? Dreaming ahead doesn't trivialize the present; it can sustain your spirit in the thick of daily tasks.

Finally, consider the legacy you're crafting: a tale of compassion, tenacity, and unwavering love. Caregiving may be forced upon you, but the grace with which you meet it is entirely yours. One day, you might look back and realize this role shaped you in profound ways—improving your empathy, forging new friendships, even guiding your life's direction. That's the hidden gift in a journey many dread. Embracing it means acknowledging both the pain and the purpose. It's not about sugarcoating reality. It's about finding meaning in each day's push and pull.

A Gentle Closing Thought

Throughout these stories of resilience, growth, joy, and perspective, a unifying message emerges: caregiving is a multi-layered experience that can break you open and then refashion you into someone stronger, more compassionate, more resourceful. Yes, it's hard. Sometimes unbearably so. But it also illuminates corners of the human heart we'd never explore otherwise. Whether you're in the early stages of adjusting to a loved one's diagnosis or a veteran in the thick of it, remember that every challenge can become a lesson, every heartbreak can be a catalyst for deeper connection.

In the next chapter, we'll shift our gaze forward—looking at future innovations, advanced planning, or perhaps the emotional transitions that come as dementia progresses further. But for now, hold tight to these inspiring tales. Let them remind you that you're not alone and that from adversity can spring transformation. In your quiet moments—maybe after tucking your loved one in or after handling a stressful phone call—reflect on the stories shared here. Know that you're part of a fellowship of caregivers around the world, each forging resilience, each finding pockets of laughter and love. And no matter how dark some days get, your story, too, holds the potential to guide and uplift someone else.

MOVING FORWARD

It's striking how much ground we've covered in these pages. We've journeyed through the essence of dementia, examined the daily trials of caregiving, explored ways to lighten burdens, protect legal rights, and nourish emotional well-being. We've listened to stories of resilience, gleaned wisdom from seasoned caregivers, and celebrated the sparks of joy that arise—even when life feels overwhelmed by confusion. Through it all, one message rings clear: you, the caregiver, are not alone.

Take a breath. Reflect. Think back on the strategies we discussed for creating a safe home environment, the validation techniques that reduce conflict, and the daily routines that ground a patient in gentle familiarity. Recall the emphasis on self-care—how vital it is to schedule your own breaks, to share responsibilities, to seek help from professionals or volunteer networks. Remember that communication is key. Whether it's non-verbal cues, calm dialogue, or mindful listening, the way you connect can soothe agitation and nurture trust. We uncovered solutions for everyday challenges, from feeding issues to wandering prevention. We delved into legal protections like Power of Attorney and advanced directives, ensuring that your loved one's voice remains heard when they can no longer advocate for themselves.

All of this was meant to empower you. As a caregiver, you deserve guidance that's both practical and emotionally supportive. My hope is that these chapters offered precisely that. Over my 25 years as a nurse in dementia care, I've witnessed how small changes in mindset or routine can revolutionize the caregiving journey. I've seen the transformative effect of communities rallying around a single family. And I've marveled at caregivers who, despite exhaustion, radiate compassion simply because they've learned to pace themselves and tap into resources. It's a humbling testament to the power of knowledge, empathy, and shared experiences.

There are some overarching takeaways worth underlining. One: *never neglect your own self-care*. This is not a trite suggestion—it's the linchpin that keeps your caregiving sustainable. Two: *communication is a bridge*, and sometimes the quietest gestures speak volumes. Three: *legal and financial preparedness* may feel daunting but offers immense peace of mind. Four: *building a support network*—whether through local community programs, online forums, or dedicated professionals—turns an isolated struggle into a collaborative effort. And five: *celebrate every small victory*. Each moment of clarity, each calm day, each new coping strategy is a stepping stone toward a more balanced life for both you and your loved one.

But caregiving doesn't stand still. Dementia is a fluid condition, shifting in waves. The needs you manage today may evolve tomorrow, requiring fresh solutions. That's why I encourage you to continue learning, adapting, and exploring. Keep reading new articles, listening to webinars, or attending support groups. Swap tips with fellow caregivers—chances are, they've tested ideas you haven't even considered. Stay open to experimenting with technology or unconventional methods. Dementia care is never one-size-fits-all, and what works well for another family might inspire your next breakthrough.

In your hands, you hold strategies and insights. Yet knowledge alone isn't enough. Action matters. Let this book spark your willingness to apply these lessons. Maybe you'll experiment with a new bedtime routine to ease sundowning or set aside fifteen minutes each morning for quick mindfulness. Perhaps you'll finally tackle the paperwork for a durable Power of Attorney or schedule a consult with a geriatric care manager. Or you'll reach out to a local volunteer group, letting them lighten your load. Every small step can amplify the quality of life you both experience.

Let's not forget gratitude. I want to thank you for your dedication—both to your loved one and to this journey of learning. Caregiving is one of the most profound acts of love and resilience, though it's often unsung. Recognize that your devotion, your willingness to wade through these pages, your quest for better care, all speak volumes about who you are. You are, without question, a vital part of someone's life, shaping their world with your patience, your presence, and your unwavering support.

As we wrap up, I'd like to point you toward a few additional resources for the road ahead:

- **The Alzheimer's Association** offers a wealth of information, hotlines, and support tools.
- **Local Area Agencies on Aging** can guide you to relevant programs, respite options, and more.
- **Online caregiver forums** (like AgingCare or the Caregiver Action Network) provide peer connection day or night.
- **Dementia-friendly communities**—seek them out, as they host events, memory cafés, and social gatherings designed for patients and caregivers alike.

Continue building your network. Expand your toolkit. And if ever in doubt, circle back to your core motivators: love, dignity, and the simple aim to make each day a touch brighter for your loved one. Even the roughest days don't negate the countless small kindnesses you offer, kindnesses that may not be verbally acknowledged but are deeply felt.

You've made it this far—through the emotional storms, the reams of paperwork, the late-night worries, and the surprising joys. No matter the challenges ahead, trust in the strength you've already shown. Lean on the tips and stories we've gathered here. Let them remind you that even when shadows lengthen, hope can flicker in unexpected corners.

Remember, you are not alone. There's a global community of caregivers forging onward, sharing your heartaches and your hopes. We are in this together, carrying the torch of empathy, forging solutions, and renewing our spirits day by day. It has been my honor to walk alongside you in these pages.

So keep going, caregiver. Keep learning, adapting, and cherishing the bond you share with the one you care for. Keep believing in the power of small victories. Keep trusting that your dedication has ripple effects far beyond what you see. Most importantly, keep remembering you have worth, strength, and an enduring compassion that stands at the heart of this entire journey.

BIBLIOGRAPHY

Below are some websites that you will find useful. I've used them for my research and also think they will be great to help you navigate your journey:

- What's the difference between ageing and dementia? https://qbi.uq.edu.au/brain/dementia/whats-difference-between-ageing-and-dementia
- Dementia Types | Symptoms, Diagnosis, Causes, Treatments https://www.alz.org/alzheimers-dementia/what-is-dementia/types-of-dementia
- 10 Early Signs and Symptoms of Alzheimer's & Dementia https://www.alz.org/alzheimers-dementia/10_signs
- Family caregivers of people with dementia - PMC https://pmc.ncbi.nlm.nih.gov/articles/PMC3181916/#:~:text=Levels%20of%20psychological%20distress%20and,larger%20when%20compared%20with%20noncaregivers.
- Alzheimer's Caregiving: Home Safety Tips https://www.nia.nih.gov/health/safety/alzheimers-caregiving-home-safety-tips
- Memory aids and tools | Alzheimer's Society https://www.alzheimers.org.uk/get-support/staying-independent/memory-aids-and-tools
- 5 Ways Tech Can Help Caregivers of Dementia Patients https://www.aarp.org/home-family/personal-technology/info-2023/dementia-caregiver-technology.html
- Community Resources - Alzheimer's & Dementia Care https://www.uclahealth.org/medical-services/geriatrics/dementia/caregiver-education/community-resources
- Non-verbal communication and dementia | Alzheimer's Society https://www.alzheimers.org.uk/about-dementia/symptoms-and-diagnosis/symptoms/non-verbal-communication-and-dementia#:~:text=Tips%20for%20non%2Dverbal%20communication,them%2C%20if%20it%20feels%20appropriate.
- Validation Therapy for Dementia: A Guide for Caregivers https://altoida.com/blog/validation-therapy-for-dementia-2/
- Sundowning: Late-day confusion https://www.mayoclinic.org/diseases-conditions/alzheimers-disease/expert-answers/sundowning/faq-20058511
- Empathy Training for Caregivers of Older People https://pubmed.ncbi.nlm.nih.gov/36148523/
- Tips for Caregivers and Families of People With Dementia https://www.alzheimers.gov/life-with-dementia/tips-caregivers
- Coping With Agitation, Aggression, and Sundowning in ... https://www.nia.nih.gov/health/alzheimers-changes-behavior-and-communication/coping-agitation-aggression-and-sundowning#:~:text=Listen%20to%20the%20person's%20concerns,10%20if%20you%20get%20upset.
- Food & Eating | Alzheimer's Association https://www.alz.org/help-support/caregiving/daily-care/food-eating
- Tools to evaluate medication management for caregivers ... https://pmc.ncbi.nlm.nih.gov/articles/PMC8483200/

- How to get power of attorney for a parent or loved one https://www.freewill.com/learn/how-to-get-power-of-attorney
- Advance Directives for Patients with Alzheimers https://www.vitas.com/hospice-and-palliative-care-basics/end-of-life-care-planning/living-wills-and-advance-directives/advance-directives-for-patients-with-alzheimers
- Financial and Legal Planning for Caregivers https://www.alz.org/help-support/caregiving/financial-legal-planning
- 9. Ethical Issues with Dementia Patients https://www.atrainceu.com/content/9-ethical-issues-dementia-patients
- Caregiver Burnout: What It Is, Symptoms & Prevention https://my.clevelandclinic.org/health/diseases/9225-caregiver-burnout
- Stress Relief Apps That Can Transform Your Life https://www.verywellmind.com/stress-relief-apps-that-can-transform-your-life-4147565
- 9 Caregiver Support Groups that Help Caregivers in Need https://www.caringbridge.org/resources/caregiver-support-groups
- The Benefits of Respite Care for Dementia Caregivers https://www.homeinstead.com/care-resources/care-planning/benefits-respite-care-dementia-caregivers/
- 6 Dementia Support Groups of 2023 - Alzheimer's https://www.verywellhealth.com/best-dementia-support-groups-4843171
- Community Resources - Alzheimer's & Dementia Care https://www.uclahealth.org/medical-services/geriatrics/dementia/caregiver-education/community-resources
- Caregiving - Alzheimer's & Dementia https://www.alz.org/help-support/caregiving
- Volunteer | Alzheimer's Association https://www.alz.org/get-involved-now/volunteer
- Caregiver Stories - CARE Registry (UCSF) https://careregistry.ucsf.edu/caregiver-stories
- Resilience in Caregivers: A Systematic Review https://pubmed.ncbi.nlm.nih.gov/31830813/
- Family Caregiving Roles and Impacts https://www.ncbi.nlm.nih.gov/books/NBK396398/
- Positive Caregiving Characteristics as a Mediator of ... https://pmc.ncbi.nlm.nih.gov/articles/PMC6262596/#:~:text=There%20is%20evidence21%E2%80%9323,more%20positive%20outlook%20on%20caregiving.

www.ingramcontent.com/pod-product-compliance
Lightning Source LLC
Chambersburg PA
CBHW071237020426
42333CB00015B/1517